Praise for *Big M*

"In the 1970's, after becoming a Jungian analyst in Zurich, I extended Jung's work and developed the Dreambody concept and Process-oriented Psychology. Dr. Pierre Morin joined me, my wife Amy, and others in exploring Process in the field of medicine and health. Illness and disease need prevention and cures—but they are also creative processes that can give us insights into who we are. Dr. Morin's *Big Medicine* is a must-read for everyone—"patients" and providers alike—who is interested in deepening the health and healing of individuals and communities."

—**Arnold Mindell**, PhD, author of *Quantum Mind*
and Healing and *The Leader's 2nd Training*

"In *Big Medicine*, Dr. Pierre Morin shows that the common conception of health as merely the proper functioning of organ systems is woefully incomplete. He reveals how our collective unity includes but transcends our chronic sense of separateness and individuality. With powerful case studies, Dr. Morin demonstrates how human health is the integration of all we are—the naughty and nice, the good and bad, warts and all. After reading *Big Medicine*, you may never think of health in the same way, and you will likely be healthier than ever before."

—**Larry Dossey**, MD, author of *One Mind: How Our Individual*
Mind Is Part of a Greater Consciousness and Why It Matters

"Dr. Morin's vision of health and healing is informed not only by his work as a medical doctor and psychological clinician, but also by his experience as a person who has heeded the Socratic call to live an 'examined life.' Defying the conventional boundaries of the individual, Dr. Morin identifies illness created by community, institutions, and the allopathic paradigm itself. This is truly a medicine for our times, one unafraid to explore the diversity in both our inner and outer landscapes."

—**David Bedrick**, JD, author of *Talking Back to Dr. Phil*:
Alternatives to Mainstream Psychology

"My experience with Dr. Morin has been a liberating one: an experience in which I have felt empowered to collaborate in my own recovery. Dr. Morin approaches his therapeutic sessions with an almost childlike sense of wonder and exploration, each "case" presenting as a miraculous individual with unique potential. I recommend *Big Medicine* for anyone aspiring to lead a meaningful life. I believe Western medical professionals would be well-served to receive this book as a blueprint for using Big Medicine to build whole humans."

—**Bill Leissner**, client

Also by

PIERRE MORIN

Inside Coma:
A New View of Awareness, Healing, and Hope
(with Gary Reiss, PhD)

Health in Sickness, Sickness in Health:
Towards a New Process Oriented Medicine

Big Medicine

TRANSFORMING YOUR RELATIONSHIP WITH YOUR BODY, HEALTH, AND COMMUNITY

Pierre Morin, MD, PhD

BELLY SONG press

Santa Fe, New Mexico

Published by:
Belly Song Press
518 Old Santa Fe Trail
Suite 1 #626
Santa Fe, NM 87505
www.bellysongpress.com

Managing Editor: Lisa Blair
Editor: Kristin Barendsen
Book cover design: David Moratto
Interior design and production: David Moratto

Printed in the United States of America on recycled paper.

Publisher's Cataloging-in-Publication Data

Morin, Pierre, 1956- author.
Big medicine : transforming your relationship with your body, health, and community / by Pierre Morin.
Santa Fe, New Mexico : Belly Song Press, [2019] |
    Includes bibliographical references and index.
ISBN: 978-0-9998094-4-0 (paperback) | 978-0-9998094-5-7 (pdf) |
    978-0-9998094-6-4 (kindle/mobipocket) | 978-0-9998094-7-1 (ePub) |
    LCCN: 2019932412
LCSH: Holistic medicine. | Medicine and psychology. |
    Mind and body. | Integrative medicine. | Self-care, Health. |
    Sick--Psychology. | Psychotherapy. | Mind and body therapies. |
    Jungian psychology. | Psychotherapy--Case studies.
LCC: R733 .M67 2019 | DDC: 610--dc23

1 3 5 7 9 10 8 6 4 2

Big Medicine

∼

TRANSFORMING YOUR RELATIONSHIP WITH YOUR BODY, HEALTH, AND COMMUNITY

CONTENTS

PREFACE

HAVING A BODY is a magical, exhilarating, and, at times, frightening experience. Being a member of a collective body such as a community can be life-affirming for some of us; yet for others it may be deadly. Medicine is the ancient art and practice of preventing harm to our individual and collective bodies and restoring their health and function.

Western medicine, however, has long been rooted in the powerful ideologies and cultural principles of individualism, colonialism, white superiority, and patriarchy. It has colluded with the abuse of the animal world and the destruction of our natural environment.[1] Also known as *allopathic medicine*, it is partly responsible for creating health disparities, has been used in multiple ways as a tool of power and control, and consistently preferences people at the center of institutionalized power while marginalizing the less privileged.

Worldwide, most people lack access to healthcare, which should be considered a fundamental human right. Our first task is to give everybody equal access to the chance to be healthy and live a meaningful life. Any additional service beyond basic care is a form of luxury and should be recognized as a privilege.

Western medicine has also brought us remarkable cures and treatments, such as immune-based cancer therapies and non-invasive surgeries.

But over the years, these approaches have disproportionally promoted the health and extended the lives of the more privileged.

Medicine, the body, emotions, psychology, and spirituality are all political issues. Whenever we focus on the individual and fail to address our societal and institutional structures, we contribute to supporting the unequal distribution of power and disparate access to resources and wellness. There is an urgent need for deep personal inquiry in support of collective change. Political and diversity consciousness are critical tools and practices for creating a more humane, equitable, and sustainable world.

I propose that we can each begin this healing and liberation work by becoming more aware and accepting of our own inner diversity.[2] Your body, the recipient of these cultural forces, is also, paradoxically, a door to understanding your own diversity and appreciating the diversity of your community. This book gives you a tool to explore your body's Dreaming and expression of diversity.

Just as our minds operate independently and most creatively during REM sleep and dreaming, our bodies have an inner intelligence that expresses itself in what we call *symptoms* or *illness*. Like artist Dreammakers in a secret studio, our minds and bodies convey messages and information that counter our notions of ourselves when we are "awake" and occupied with living our external lives. In the alternate reality of night dreams, in the altered states between dreaming and wakefulness, and through our bodies' obscure intelligence, we can experience creative insights and spiritual revelations. They can help us understand our deeper selves and our inner diversity. Used well, they can contribute to building community, social, and systemic change.

In this book, my own inner diversity will express itself in varying voices. My passionate advocacy self, my compassionate emotional side, my measured intellectual mind, and my eldership voice will appear at different points across the pages and might at times create confusion and contradiction. As a white, cisgender, straight, and financially secure man, I can't escape the mainstream cultural currents. My socialization into these specific frames of references will seep into the views and opinions that I express here and will undeniably show my biases. The topics that I speak to are unresolved group processes that no one voice or one author can duly capture. They will need your involvement as I need your feedback. I hope that I will be humble enough to accept it graciously.

Portland, August 2018

ACKNOWLEDGMENTS

⁓

THE FIRST SEEDS of this book were sown 35 years ago at a serendipitous meeting in Basel, Switzerland. At a gathering of friends, I met Arnold Mindell, founder of process-oriented psychology. He shared with us his new and revolutionary approach to working with body symptoms.

I had just finished medical school, and at first I was taken aback by a psychology that appeared to question the very foundation of medicine: its notion of pathology. But Arny's uncanny creative spirit and mind, and his radical reframing of my profession, launched me on a journey to study process-oriented psychology and move to the United States.

On the Oregon coast, I participated in the original Lava Rock clinics, which formed the inspiration for this book. They were led by Arny and Amy Mindell and Ellen and Max Schupach, the ingenious minds behind this work. In these weeklong clinics, people with chronic illnesses joined a community of providers to explore the stories and meanings that body symptoms entail. These clinics started me on a path of inquiry into the dreaming world of physical symptoms, health, and sickness.

I am thankful to Kara Wilde, Emetchi, and Dr. Jai Tomlin, the colleagues with whom I facilitate monthly Dreambody Medicine Forums in Portland. These forums have served as rich grounds for my research and practice of Big Medicine. Many of the stories in this book originated in these forums.

Though he is no longer alive, I must thank Friedrich Nietzsche, who coined the term *Grosse Gesundheit*. His struggle with chronic illness spurred him to challenge conventional notions of health. He offered an expanded view of healing that includes sickness as a heroes' rite of passage toward a bigger health.

Our world is experiencing an unparalleled level of displacement, with refugees fleeing conflicts in record numbers. My own ancestors were Moors and Huguenots who fled Spain and France because of religious persecution. I'm grateful that for the past 15 years, I've had the opportunity to help refugees resettle in Oregon. Every day, they show me the extraordinary resilience of the human spirit and body. These refugees are my teachers, and their stories of trauma and hope both inspire and humble me. They have also awakened me to the increasing health disparities in our society and the need for medicine to advocate for health as a human right.

I would like to thank my friend and mentor Max Schupach for his continuous support and belief in me. He helped me overcome my doubts about writing, and he published my first book, *Health in Sickness, Sickness in Health.*

Many thanks to my editor, Kristin Barendsen; her sensitive corrections and precise feedback gave me the confidence to continue writing. My managing editors and publishers, Lisa Blair and David Bedrick of Belly Song Press, gave me much constructive feedback and encouragement. Thanks to them, this book improved immensely. My colleagues Bill Say and Lane Arye read drafts of chapters that relate to community health and social justice. Their remarks led me to deepen my understanding of rank and power dynamics as well as concerns of equity and inclusion.

My wife, Kara Wilde, surrounded me with love and support. She gave me the space to spend hours in my own creative world, and she helped brainstorm many of the ideas that are embedded in this book. Her empathic and artistic spirit is a bottomless source of love, inspiration, and companionship. My son Jem created the graphs in this book.

Finally, I would like to dedicate this book to all the individuals who entrusted me with their stories of injury, illness, health, and healing. By seeking wellness and meaning within and beyond their trauma and sickness, they are the true pioneers of Big Medicine.

INTRODUCTION

LINNEA, A FIERY red-haired Scott, is literally burning. Her skin is on fire. She has suffered since her early childhood from chronic atopic eczema. As a baby, she was cranky and colicky and couldn't tolerate cow's milk. Her life is an endless litany of doctor's visits—nightmares of needles puncturing her skin hoping to desensitize her body to the attacking allergens. She almost resented giving birth to her daughter because her pregnancy was the only respite she'd experienced from the constant itchy flares that make her scratch her skin raw and bloody.

But with help from her coach, she enters the world of the burning flame, becomes the blaze that lifts and dissipates in flowing motions into the sky. On that journey, she shrieks with anger and passion, transforms into smoke, and liberates herself from her earthly body to join Nature,[3] who calls her to advocate for her more forcefully.

Linnea presents with all the typical medical symptoms, genetic attributes, and grueling illness narratives of someone with severe chronic eczema, a condition that conventional medicine has few remedies for. Patients like Linnea run from one medical professional to another and succumb again and again to the burning skin flares. They become discouraged and get depressed, and some even think of suicide as a way out of the relentless bad dream.

This book offers an alternative way of thinking about health, disease, and medicine *and will transform your relationship with your body.* I call this approach *Big Medicine,* in contrast to *small medicine,* or mainstream Western medicine. For Linnea, Big Medicine meant to embrace the burning, explore its world, and discover a renewed purpose as an ambassador for Nature. Her lifelong struggles with chronic illness have led her to moments of despair and depression but finally also allowed her to dive deeply into her own being and find a new sense of self. Big Medicine doesn't replace all the benefits of small medicine. Rather, it is an invitation to also uncover the embodied mind and resourcefulness that comes from the body's lived experience even when small medicine says we have a disease and asks us to reject it.

Big Medicine continues the inquiry into health that I began with my book *Health in Sickness, Sickness in Health.*[4] The latter proposes that there are valuable aspects to sickness, and that our concepts of health have problematic side effects that add a burden of suffering. I concluded *Health in Sickness* with a new definition of health that I called, in alignment with the German philosopher Nietzsche, *grosse Gesundheit,* or *Big Health.* Big Health is an awareness approach to health and sickness that facilitates all facets of someone's experience in a holistic way, including the community and social ones.

With *Big Medicine,* I am deepening the conversation to explore medicine and "healing" in a radical new way that starts with the core subjective experience of feeling sick and follows the process in which sickness is embedded. (For Linnea, this is feeling the burning sensation, embodying the flame, transforming into its smoke, etc.) *Big Medicine* explores the current mainstream topography of health and illness and lays out the foundation of a new holistic and non-pathologizing approach to venturing through the experience of illness—one that is informed by process-oriented psychology. I then discuss Process, the science of inner experiences, and the practice of presence. As the journey continues, I look at relationships and communities both as medicine and as creators of sickness. I conclude by advocating for a new colorful, communal fabric of health, medicine, and healing.

My most ardent wish is for you, the reader, to find some insights about your own path and processes. If you are a patient, I want to help you develop an attitude toward your health that values all medical approaches and the need for diagnosis and treatment whenever necessary. In addition, I want to offer you a new way of exploring illness that does not pathologize it—one that is interested in the deeper wisdom that lies hidden underneath the bedrock of disease, pain, and suffering. If you are a healthcare provider, I want to stimulate you to think of health in a non-dual, holistic way and give you tools that will help you facilitate your clients' journeys through illness toward true healing.

The Origins of Big Medicine

Today's version of medicine, what I call *small medicine*, has lost its art. It has turned into the provision of healthcare, which has morphed into a practice that is dominated by technologies, process flow charts, decision trees, and lists of best practices. It is based on the idea that the body is a machine built as a collection of machines. Healthcare supplies the mechanics that repair the failing or broken machine. This version of medicine is very powerful and often successful; we still need to use it. But medicine has lost its depth, art, and soul, as well as its human and social connection.

I began to form the concept of Big Medicine as a young resident just out of medical school, after responding to an invitation from my physician friend Martin Vosseler. Martin was an unconventional doctor, in many ways like the American physician, comedian, and social activist Patch Adams, who founded the Gesundheit Institute in 1971.

Martin had a one-man private practice on the Rhine border in Basel. As part of his medical practice, he invited a person of interest to speak each month, such as a politician, poet, environmentalist, or social activist. They would share their views and practices and we, the invited circle of friends, would discuss how these ideas could inform our lives and medical practices.

One evening, he invited Arnold Mindell, the founder of process-oriented psychology, to demonstrate his uncanny approach to body symptoms. Martin volunteered to explore his own symptoms of repetitive strain injury (RSI), and 35 years later, I still vividly remember the fascination I felt as I witnessed Arny unveiling the story and process, the depth and meaning that lay beneath what medically was an uncomplicated condition that would probably resolve easily with some rest.

Many years later, Martin told me how life-changing this experience had been for him. His RSI had stemmed from filling thousands of envelopes with political leaflets. Arny helped Martin unfold the pain in his hand, which required him to stop in his tracks, rest, and re-examine the scope of his involvement in medicine, relationships, and political action. This experience spurred Martin to eventually leave medicine and devote his life to environmental activism.

This represented a paradigm shift for me. A body experience was not only a nuisance or a symptom of something broken that needed to be fixed. It had its own relevance that was deeply embedded in Martin's history, personality, current life situation, and aspirations. Big Medicine started that evening and has evolved through my 35 years of studies in process-oriented psychology and medicine.

The first seminar in process-oriented psychology I attended after that watershed night was a seminar on group dynamics and conflict resolution led by Arnold Mindell. It was a five-day seminar in Tschierv, a remote village in the Swiss Alps. We were about 45 participants all staying under the same roof in a big Swiss mountain cabin and working together on issues within our group, such as gender and class. There was also one African-American woman who brought race to the forefront, an issue that was, in those days, little spoken about in Switzerland. The interactions were wild, intense, and transformational. I remember glass shattering and people screaming and running out into the Alpine meadows.

Medicine, at that time, tended to attract shy, introverted, and conforming individuals into its studies and practice, and I was one of them. The group dynamics I witnessed in Tschierv were deeply disturbing to me, but I stayed and survived. The experience sparked in me a curiosity about the social and community aspects of medicine that later led to my doctoral studies in social medicine and health psychology. In these studies, I learned about the injustices of our social arrangements that create health disparities. Thus, individual health and community health are the two pillars of my version of medicine.

How to Read This Book

Big Medicine is meant to inspire your thinking and stimulate self-reflection. To complement the insights and anecdotes in each chapter, I give some coaching guidance in the form of inner work exercises. In this way, you can use it as a self-help book. If you are a patient, please use the exercises along with your own common sense and intuition, and consult with your health providers. If you are a provider, you can use the exercises to learn more about yourself and to find new creative and Process-informed ways you can assist your clients and patients.

As illustrations, I rely on examples from my own experience and on stories from people I have coached and counseled. While they have consented to have their stories published, I have kept their demographic information private and changed their names.

I begin by sharing my personal perspective on health. I discuss some features of small medicine, or what I call *bell curve medicine,* and contrast them with concepts of Big Health and Big Medicine. After exploring the wisdom of inner experiences through the lens of process-oriented psychology, I delve into the practice of presence—the source of Big Medicine's healing powers. This all leads to an examination of how we can use the Big Medicine paradigm—not only in our individual lives, but also in our relationships with others and our communities.

Chapter 1

The Landscape of Health, Medicine, and Healing

～2～

O N NOVEMBER 7, 2016, the poet and singer Leonard Cohen passed on. The chorus of my favorite Leonard Cohen song, "Anthem," goes like this: "Ring the bells that still can ring; forget your perfect offering; there is a crack, a crack in everything; that's how the light gets in." In my book *Health in Sickness, Sickness in Health,* I shared these lines as a metaphor for valuing our imperfections and "cracks." Cracks are where light gets in, where awareness can emerge. Could there be some value to the cracks in our health—that is, our illnesses? The upset of a disease, I explained in the book, is an overture for a new understanding and learning. Thus, health in sickness.

As an immigrant from Switzerland with English as my third language, I work in a very diverse environment helping refugees resettle in the United States. I am passionate about medicine and the world. My loving uncle Pierre Girard was an acclaimed doctor, but a mountain farmer and vintner at heart. He inspired me to study medicine. Although I am not currently working as a medical doctor, I have served as such in the past in various mainstream medical settings.

Health, medicine, and healing have been my central professional focus for the past 45 years. I have experienced the benefits of Western medicine up close. But I have also seen the limitations of Western medicine, how its benefits are unequally distributed, how most medical interventions treat the individual and ignore their family and community, and how our narrow emphasis on health marginalizes so many aspects of our lives. My perspective changed after Arnold Mindell introduced me to his radical paradigm shift around body symptoms, medicine, and health. This encounter led me to transition my work from mainstream medicine into counseling, coaching, and consulting with individuals and groups, employing the methods of process-oriented psychology and Big Medicine.

Throughout my conventional medical career, never did I learn that illness could be anything other than an enemy, much less an opportunity for growth and heightened awareness.

Thus, I am excited to present you with my unique and very personal perspective on the landscape of health, medicine, and healing. Big Medicine draws on the theories and concepts of process-oriented psychology, which was developed by Arny and Amy Mindell and their colleagues. In this book, I will share my own journey and bring a distinctive note to the topic. I will first lay out the mainstream thinking of health and illness, and then contrast them with my own viewpoints, which I draw from process-oriented psychology.

Also known as "Process Work," process-oriented psychology views every experience as one worth exploring to uncover its potential for new learning and meaning. Its approach is strictly non-pathological, which allows us as patients and providers to shift our mindset and begin to see ill health as more than disease.

With Big Medicine, I make the case that health has been elevated to the dominant culture of our experience and that disease has been relegated to refugee status. We marginalize disease and illness as foreign and try to keep them out as best we can. We exclude the language and culture of disease from our notion of health. In Big Medicine, disease is not only failed health but also a new cultural experience that has its own language and meaning.

Some Definitions

Before I continue, let me in broad strokes explain some of the concepts I will use throughout the book. I will detail the definitions in later chapters. *Health* is a theoretical construct that describes an ideal state of your body and mind. As we will see, that ideal state is actually a fallacy that adds a layer of suffering for those who experience ill health. I define health as a theory and *medicine* as the application of health sciences for the purposes of *healing*. For example, in my case, health is an idea of a state without asthma, and medicine is the use of my asthma inhaler to get relief.

Small health is a term that stresses the reductionist and mechanistic features of mainstream Western or allopathic medicine. In Chapter 2, I discuss the *bell curve model of health*, which highlights the normative elements of small health. *Big Health*, as stated earlier, endorses a more inclusive concept of health—one that sees disease and illness as a path toward health. *Big Medicine* is my take on a multi-layered, holistic approach to healing that is based on Big Health concepts.

Big Medicine is the application of Big Health. In addition, Big Medicine uses theories and methods from process-oriented psychology to explore and facilitate a person's and community's experiences of health and sickness. Big Medicine is *Process-informed,* as it highlights the dynamic, forward-moving qualities of life and looks at the manifestations of life with a value-neutral ethical lens.

Small health and medicine see the body as a complex machine that needs maintenance to remain tuned and repair when it's broken. Symptoms are indicators that something is wrong; they help health professionals identify which parts are malfunctioning or broken. Medications, surgeries, and other interventions are tools for fixing the problems. Secondary to all of this are the body's owner, his or her psychology, and the environment and community he or she lives in. These factors are rarely addressed as part of the health issue. If at all, the social, emotional, and psychological aspects of ill health are referred to social workers and counselors—healthcare providers who have less status than their physical health counterparts and who are poorly compensated for their services. The dominance of small health thinking and values is maintained by ingrained political and economic structures that protect the profits of the corporate health industry.

Health is a complex and multi-layered story. It is a figment of our imagination, an ideal that may not be helpful any longer. Or better, we need to rethink the concept of health and find new modes of relating to all the existential processes that surround our notion of health. I want to suggest a way we can retake ownership of our bodies, the experiences they present us with, and our community relationships around health.

For this purpose, I propose to differentiate between small health and medicine and Big Health and Medicine. Small health and medicine are the conventional approaches. For Linnea, my client with eczema, these approaches included avoiding cow's milk and other foods; enduring many harrowing courses of desensitization to allergens; treating the symptoms with antibiotics, cortisone, and an array of topical ointments; and trying acupuncture, homeopathy, and several other modalities. Such treatments are invaluable, and, as we will see, problematic. They confined Linnea into the identity of a diseased person: someone who is not whole, someone who (besides enduring the excruciating pain) must hide her body and its rashes.

Big Health and Medicine accept the need for small health and medicine, but combine it with a new Process-informed approach that places each individual and community at the center. Our inner experiences and personal stories are the backbone of this new approach. In small medicine, our subjective knowledge has been disenfranchised in favor of objective test results. Big Medicine reintegrates the psychological and emotional know-how of us as individuals and communities.

In mainstream culture, health has a dominant and favored standing. The majority perspective turns against illness, disease, and (ultimately) death. This makes good sense. Nobody in their right mind wants to fall ill, suffer, and die. It doesn't seem right to embrace disease. On the other hand, we have no choice. Ill health and death are part of the fabric of life. Why not then be curious, learn a new language, and discover a new landscape and culture? Big Medicine aims to take you on a journey that will help you deepen your grasp of the diverse and multifaceted manifestations of your being. Over time, this will include drifting through health and pausing at disease. Getting to know a symptom is like traveling to a foreign country. Some of its manifestations are difficult, while others open up new insights and perspectives.

Culture and Health

Culture not only shapes our attitude toward health, illness, and death —it also contributes to the burden of disease. Cultural structures of systemic oppression, including racism, sexism, and classism, create physiological stress that translates into disease and adds to health disparities. The politics and policies of governments that support unequal sharing of resources and opportunities foster marginalization and create a more discriminatory distribution of disease. In this way, politics and policies are directly linked to life expectancies and our individual likelihood of staying healthy. Cultural, psychosocial, and psychopolitical forces can actually influence our physiologies and the metabolisms of our bodies by causing, for example, trauma, stress, tension, anxiety, and depression.[5]

Diseases, from a Process-informed perspective, express marginalized aspects of our identity. These marginalized aspects embrace a diverse set of values and beliefs, creating (in a way) their own culture. In addition, community relationships can help keep us healthy or make us sick. Big Medicine therefore uses a cultural lens to better understand our illness experience and the systemic structures that affect our bodies and minds. Life is a playground in which health and illness coexist. In Big Medicine, both are seen as an articulation of a deeper Process that is present in individual and communal experiences.

In Western culture, we think that to be normal is to be healthy. The media floods us with information and images of idealized young, healthy, and immortal bodies. We assign doctors, chiropractors, naturopaths, psychologists, and fitness trainers with the responsibility to keep us healthy, and we blame them if they don't succeed. And cultural ideas about health—such as norms for fitness levels, weight, and body size—are used constantly to privilege some people over others. What is going on?

The Israeli sociologist Aaron Antonovsky said, "People are as good as dead, yet need to live."[6] He studied how some Jews survived the Holocaust and the resettlement to Israel, two of the most stressful experiences imaginable. While not everybody faces such major perils, we all live with a body that is under the constant threat of getting injured or sick, and the everyday miracle is that we don't succumb to the dangers and diseases that surround us. As we continually encounter potential health hazards, our bodies adjust. These health threats are heightened by our constitutional factors, lifestyle habits, and community dynamics. Thankfully, we sleepwalk most of the time through these risks. It would overwhelm us to understand all the dangers we face each day. And the self-protective and self-healing abilities of our bodies and minds are truly extraordinary.

But then, many of us live with chronic illness—and as we age, our failing health becomes a reality we all must face. By marginalizing illness and death, we create a culture that is obsessed with small health and preventing death for as long as possible. This attitude, albeit sensible in some ways, limits our psychological and spiritual growth and creates a refugee problem for people who are less fortunate in their ability to stay healthy and overcome the challenges of disease and aging. We treat our illnesses as displaced aspects of ourselves and feel exiled from the rest of the community.

A Car Accident and Big Medicine

The following story is an example of using Big Medicine to help a client overcome the trauma of an accident and its devastating consequences. With my wife and two other colleagues, I facilitate a monthly Dream-body Medicine forum.[7] These forums consist of two-hour meetings in which we study, in a small group setting, the subjective disease experience of an individual and its relevance for the group and community.

In this context, I recently coached Martha, a successful middle-aged professional who had experienced two serious car accidents about one year apart. In the first accident, while Martha was driving down a highway, the cab of an 18-wheeler semi- in the middle lane suddenly swerved into Martha's lane with no warning. The collision propelled her car, spinning, across several lanes until it crashed into the side railing. Martha is not sure if she hit her head, but the spinning forces caused some shearing of brain tissue and other secondary injuries to her kidneys and shoulders.

Her recovery included multiple surgeries and rehabilitative therapies. Over time, she slowly improved from the debilitating daily headaches, mental fuzziness, and confusion caused by the brain injury. Understandably, Martha remained very anxious about driving, and she had a persistent feeling that she would be in an accident again.

And indeed, this is what happened two weeks before I worked with her. She was riding in the back of a taxi when she saw a car coming toward her head. She barely had time to pull her arms up to protect her head. Thankfully, the side airbag deployed and prevented Martha from getting seriously injured. Nevertheless, she experienced a second concussion, which set back her recovery.

In the exploration we did together, Martha was mostly interested in learning more about the impact of the car that had hit her. The concussion had left her feeling low, fatigued and upset about the loss of her identity as a competent, energetic businesswoman.

I proposed that she watch myself and a colleague re-enact the

accident. I played Martha sitting in the back of the taxi, and my colleague played the car that hit her. Her job was to watch us and intervene
whenever she felt like it—or not. While I was role-playing her, I had the
intuition to verbally attack the car that was going to hit me. I started
yelling at the incoming car to back off and leave me alone. Martha,
watching me, started laughing and encouraging me. I asked her to join
me in confronting the power that was going to hit her. A loud, forceful
interaction ensued between her and the "car."

Later, Martha stepped into the role of the car and explored the
message that the "car" might be trying to wake her up to. As the car, she
challenged herself to believe in her talents and power. In this interaction, she managed to temporarily overcome the sense of being victimized by the car that hit her and reconnect with her innate strength and
competence.

As a group, we then discussed the social dynamics that affect wom-
en's and men's sense of empowerment and competence, how we respond
to trauma and victimization, and how as a community we project power onto institutions and individuals that hold high social rank, such as
the police, government actors, and big business and organizations.
Often, we externalize power and remain invested in being a victim
because we would rather blame the powerful for the harm we experience than step into our own power.

Weeks later, I was able to coach Martha again. This time, she asked
to focus on some incapacitating stabbing pains and dull aches she had
been experiencing since the second car accident. The throbbing was
keeping her from sleeping at night. She helped me re-create the subjective pain experience. With my co-facilitator, we helped her give the
"pain maker" a voice.

In a role play, my colleague and I asked Martha how we could best
step into what was creating her pain in that moment. Alternating between the role of the one who experiences the pain and the one who
manifests the pain, we slowly uncovered in the pain maker a powerful
voice that challenged Martha to stay awake and to believe more in the

impact she could have in the world. Very comparable to her process weeks earlier, the car that hit her and the pain that kept her awake were "demanding" to be heard—and their message was that she needed to step more into her own power and have more impact in the world.

The group picked up on this theme, and each of us spoke about how we sometimes shy away from believing in ourselves and what we can bring to the community.

Small health and medicine focus on treating physical injuries and facilitating the recovery process. In Martha's case, they helped her rehabilitate from the effects of the accidents. Big Health and Medicine help us more deeply inquire into the psychological and existential aspects of health challenges. Using Process-informed methods, Big Medicine helps us gain a more holistic view of health that paradoxically includes the illness or injury experience as a means to a larger understanding of ourselves and our communities. For Martha and the group that witnessed her Process, the Big Medicine approach gave a window into how to negotiate issues of trauma, pain, power, and competence.

Koubanao — My Introduction to Big Medicine

This is a personal story. In hindsight, it was my first confrontation and lived experience with Big Medicine. At that time, I didn't know, I was too engrossed in learning the ropes of small medicine. As a newly graduated doctor living in Basel, Switzerland, where I had spent my entire life, I was looking for residency placements. It was the 1980s. I had completed my medical studies, my internship rotations, and one year as a resident in family medicine. One day I saw a notice in a medical journal that a Swiss-Italian nonprofit was looking for a doctor to operate a rural hospital in Koubanao, a village in the south of Senegal. The mystique of the village name and the adventure I associated with Africa lured me into applying. I flew there to explore the location, the people, and the job I would be performing.

It was at the end of the dry season, and everything appeared as romantic as I had imagined it. I fell in love with the place and the people and accepted the position. Three months later, in the middle of the rainy season, I returned with my partner to begin my work assignment. Our lodging was a brick house that previous expatriates had built. It was at the edge of the forest and isolated from the village —which was a mile further up the hill. There were only a few huts close by that were occupied by some Bantu people, whom we soon learned were marginalized from the rest of the community.

This whole setup felt strange. I had seen the house in my previous scouting visit and had talked to my predecessor, an Africa-savvy Swiss doctor, who was inhabiting it. At that time, nothing had appeared abnormal. On the contrary, the location and surroundings had seemed idyllic, and the forest provided welcome shade. With the change in season, my experience and judgment shifted. This change began at dusk, when suddenly we were invaded by mosquitos that thrived in the breeding grounds of the now rainy forest. Nothing repelled them; they were everywhere. We hurried through dinner, choking on the fumes of the mosquito coils burning under our table. Barely able to eat, we dove under the mosquito nets on our bed and then spent hours hunting the mosquitos that had managed to squeeze below the net as we entered the hoped-for shelter. It was a nightmare.

I now understood why only the banned Bantu families were living close by. No one who knew the local climate would build a dwelling in this area. Some previous aid developers had chosen this spot for their housing during the dry season, ignoring the villagers' warnings.

Within two weeks, my partner and I—along with another Swiss expatriate couple and their three-year-old child—fell sick with fever, chills, and headaches. I immediately suspected malaria, but we were all taking Chloroquine to prevent us from getting it. What had happened? There were no reports of Chloroquine-resistant malaria strains in West Africa. But the blood smears I took from all five of us showed malaria parasites. Despite the denial of local experts, I suspected that we were experiencing the advent of the first resistant strains, and I started us on medication that would treat that resistant type of malaria.

I had only a few doses of the appropriate medication with me— enough to treat only four of us. Additionally, I had one course of another newer and still experimental medication (Lariam), which I took to treat myself. Seeing that we were all slow to respond to the treatment, I decided to evacuate us to Ziguinchor, the nearest city that had a regional hospital and an airport, in case we needed more intensive support. We were able to stay at a friend's house, which gave us some respite.

Coincidentally, the region was also experiencing a cholera epidemic, and the hospital was becoming unsafe, with all the patients in need of hydration and antibiotic treatment flocking to it and overwhelming the clinical staff's capacity to handle the situation. As the sun set and the tropical night rose, the women of Ziguinchor gathered, drumming and chanting through the streets in an attempt to scare the cholera spirits away. I was lying in bed with a high fever listening to these exotic and chilling sounds. I drifted in and out of dreams, haunted by the beats of the drums and the rhythms of the incanting voices.

The friend who was hosting us recommended that we transfer to Senegal's capital, Dakar, which required us to take a plane that flew only twice a day. Despite a rush of people trying to flee from the cholera and get tickets, we were able to board the second plane. It was a small plane seating about 30 people. It taxied to the end of the runway and then stopped. The pilot informed us that another sick passenger on a stretcher had to board, which meant that some of us had to give up their space and return to the gate. I panicked, fearing we would be chosen, but fortunately for us, our status and light skin saved us. We spent a grueling two-hour flight in the company of a very sick African elder and panicking that we would catch his cholera on top of having malaria.

In Dakar, we received more medical tests that remained inconclusive. I continued my course of Lariam. That night in a hotel room, I started developing side effects to this new experimental drug. I became delirious and psychotic. Inexplicably, my body started feeling alien, not part of me. I kept touching my legs in an effort to connect with my body. It had become an object that I could not relate to anymore. I was merely a thought or spirit, dissociated from any material reality. Intermittently, I still had some awareness that this perception was drug-induced, which gave me some comfort—but nevertheless, this experience was extremely distressing and scary.

A few years earlier, on an extended trip to Mexico, I had visited a curandero who swayed a raw egg over my body to capture the essence of my ailments. He cracked it open, read the contents, and gave me all sorts of insights. Now in my delirium, I had fixating thoughts that only a shaman and traditional healer could help me. It was late at night. My conviction compelled me to feverishly dress and stagger toward the stairs to roam the city's night streets in search of this imagined savior. My partner was a psychiatric nurse, herself still recovering from malaria. She stopped me from leaving the hotel and dragged me into a cold shower to shock me back into consciousness and reality. Somehow, we got through the night and were able to get to Dakar's international airport, where a Swiss medevac plane waited for us.

Back in Switzerland, serological tests confirmed my diagnosis of Chloroquine-resistant malaria. The Lariam treatment slowly became effective, and the side effects subsided as well. After some recovery time, I returned to Koubanao, which in the meantime had returned to the beauty and safety of the dry season. Thankfully, I never experienced such an extreme state again.

The shaman, though, stayed with me. Over the years, my impulse to seek the help of a shaman, as dangerous as it was in the specific context of that night in Dakar, has acquired some truth and meaning for me. In my psychosis, I was on to something important. This was my first encounter with serious illness. Besides initiating me into what it means to be sick and a patient, my disembodied and dissociated state awakened me to the importance of another world and reality, one more dreamlike and spirited—a world that shaman, priests, and meditators of all sorts have visited for centuries. In my extreme state, I was becoming a shaman who was liberating himself from the material body to get in touch with another realm and reality. The "shaman" is an aspect of myself that attempted to break through in a crisis. It goes against my Swiss upbringing, my routine tendency to favor practical and rational aspects of life, and my task-oriented approach to living. Despite the help of many coaches and therapists, I continue to have difficulties integrating this aspect of myself. But this Process taught me to follow my inner experiences and use them for the benefit of myself and my patients.

More than 30 years after this initial crisis-mediated introduction to my own shamanic nature, I have become more and more aware of its relevance, and it motivates me to delve into the spiritual dimensions of Big Medicine (see Chapters 5, 7, and 10).

Dreaming and Big Medicine

Night dreams are usually not connected to health and body symptoms. Conventional thinking says that dreams cannot predict health symptoms. On the other hand, if you closely follow someone's subjective body sensations, they will often associate these experiences with recent night dreams that share related qualities. For example, after a gallbladder surgery I had several years ago because of an inflamed gallstone, I experienced some complications due to a blockage in my bile duct. The abdominal cramping I felt was like a tight vise. The surgeon recommended a second surgery. That night, I dreamed of a chimney that was letting out a lot of steam, and in the morning my pre-operative check showed that the blockage was gone.

Another interesting dream illustrates the connection between dreaming and Big Medicine and the subjective intelligence that dreams can have. Jeon, a Korean student of process-oriented psychology, dreamed she was taking a class led by a certain famous obstetrician who had inspired her in waking life. In her dream, as she was participating in the class activities, the sun began to eclipse, which put everybody in a state of awe.

As the dream continued, the physician teacher handed Jeon a small silver stag beetle. He told her that the beetle was precious and unique and asked her to take good care of it and help it grow. In her dream, she wondered how to do that and woke up. From the dream, she took that she was pregnant, which turned out to be true.

Jeon associated the solar eclipse with a man and a woman coming together. She explained that the Korean word for stag beetle also has connotations of softness and femininity, and that silver is usually associated with female qualities. Jeon felt that she was asked to carry the physician's legacy, which encompassed the merging of the sun and moon. Jeon also felt encouraged to trust her inner knowing and overcome her shyness about her ability to perceive things without direct sensory experience.

The baby whom she carried and gave birth to nine months later turned out to be a girl. What an amazing dream! What created the dream, and how did the not-yet-conscious pregnancy influence the dream? Where does that inner knowledge come from? Who or what is the Dreammaker; who is creating this web of non-local connections?

Big Medicine builds on objective, factual, and scientific knowledge as well as on inner subjective intelligence, which is harder to grasp and trust. We can't gain access to this inner knowing through our normal sensory perceptions. It is present and available through other means of knowing. That knowing appears to be transpersonal and non-local, across time and space. It is numinous and synchronistic. Many names have been given to these types of experiences: the Tao, God, the universe, Process Mind, and more.

In Big Medicine, illness is both a physical reality and a dream that is connected to our inner subjective lives. It has real material consequences that require small health attention and inner significance that is revealed through the science of inner truth.

Big Medicine acknowledges the value of bringing inner empirical knowledge into medicine and our personal lives. To cure my malaria, I relied on the outer empirical knowledge of medicine as a science, one that has its roots in the schools that excluded the ancient shamans and "charlatans" to focus on experimentally supported facts. I am not proposing that we go back in time. But I think that now is the moment to take the next evolutionary step toward a new medicine and open ourselves to the value and meaning of our subjective experiences (Big Health). In this way, we can honor the timeless knowledge of inner truth, while at the same time respecting outer, observable, and measurable truths.

In modern times, we have become quite adept at understanding the knowledge we draw from outer empirical facts—knowledge we access through our outwardly oriented senses. Rightfully, we question the validity of beliefs and assumptions that are based on inner subjective experiences. We see the polarization that results from some faith-based convictions and retreat to what we perceive as more reliable and objective evidence. But in so doing, we contribute to marginalizing centuries-old spiritual wisdom, shamanic traditions, and Indigenous practices that access a reality beyond the boundaries of our senses—a reality that dwells within the inner recesses of our subjective worlds and that is in communion with the natural world. Big Medicine is an invitation to stop and listen to our subjective states and the science-based medical knowledge they complement.

My delusion to seek healing from a shaman, Jeon's revelatory dream, and my client's car accident and chronic pain: Do we put them aside as quirks of our minds, as entertaining curiosities that have no real significance? Or do we take them as opportunities to study a parallel inner truth that complements the outer scientific actuality? Big Medicine is an attempt to bridge these two worlds; it is a journey of rediscovering our inner lives and stepping forward on a more meaningful path.

Chapter 2

THE BELL CURVE MODEL
OF HEALTH AND MEDICINE

IMAGINE THAT you are lying on a doctor's examination table, wearing just your underwear and a loose patient's robe that leaves you barely protected and amplifies your feeling of vulnerability. The doctor comes in with the test results you have been anticipating for more than a week. He gives you his verdict. Either you fall inside or outside the range of normality and health.

And if the results are not good, you immediately sense that you've been thrown out of your previously familiar territory of health and normality. Your doctor's demeanor changes, and everybody around you suddenly treats you differently. With one test result, everything can change. You feel like a different person, and your family and friends approach you as if you might die next week. What is going on?

Conventional medicine uses normal distribution or bell curves to determine what we view as healthy and normal. It compares our individual health markers to statistical norms to see if they deviate or conform. While deviations help us define what is "normal," this process shapes our experience of our own health and makes us feel marginalized, expelled from the land of health, and inferior if we don't fit inside the bell curve.

Big Medicine, in contrast, values the outlier experiences as much as those that fit within the bell curve. It rejects the narrow duality of health and sickness in favor of a Process-informed perspective that explores our experience, be it of so-called "health" or "sickness."

Bell Curve Medicine

How we define health and disease and the way we frame the understanding of these concepts have important social and cultural significance. On a societal level, the definitions of the terms *health* and *disease* influence healthcare policies such as access to medical care, what is considered a disability that is eligible for social support benefits, how research funds are allocated, and more. On an interpersonal level, our conventional but insensitive use of these terms creates barriers and divisions. When we separate the diseased from the healthy, we pathologize individuals and groups who are unwell.

Most medical professionals and laypeople alike believe that a person is healthy if he or she has no disease. The logic goes like this: Health is normal functioning in the absence of disease. Disease and injury are objective physiological conditions that lead to the disruption of normal functioning. And health and normal functioning are considered to be the standard experiences that most people have.

Thus, *health* becomes the norm based on which any aberrant experience gets classified as *disease* or *impairment*. The term *disease* conventionally describes the objective physiological malfunctions, whereas *illness* or *sickness* are used to stress the subjective experiences or symptoms that result from these objective breakdowns. *Illness* also includes the social attributions and judgments that come with the experience and impairment. Finally, *disability* refers to the social consequences of the impairment.

I have a client who was recently diagnosed with cervical cancer. Some of the cells in her cervix have turned malignant. Physicians use various criteria to evaluate the cells' level of malignancy, the size of the tumor or the volume of cells turned malignant, and the malignant cells' behavior in the surrounding environment. All of the objective qualities and behaviors of the cells allow physicians to determine the stage of the cancer and how far away from normality and health the tumor is.

The impairment is the mixture of experiences my client has because of the cancer: The fear and anxiety it produces, the time it takes her away from living her normal life, and the possible consequences and side effects of treatments she might pursue.

The cancer was discovered because my client had a probably unrelated inflammation of the bladder, which caused her some pain and discomfort. The cancer is not yet causing her any direct subjective symptoms or illness. So at this point, the illness is manifesting as the distress and fear she feels about what could happen and by the decrease in femininity that could be a side effect of some treatments. My client would probably feel disabled if she were to suffer long-lasting effects from a surgical intervention, such as incontinence. She would enter a more formal state of disability if she were forced to stop working and needed financial support such as Social Security benefits.

The "Normal" Distribution of Health

The frequency and normal distribution of experiences determine what medical science considers to be health norms. The graphic illustration of this statistical distribution of health is a bell-shaped curve. Under the bell is the delineated sector that entails the health norm. Outside of the bell curve are the statistical outliers that are called *disease*.

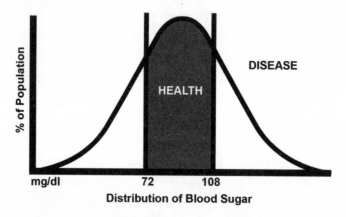

Figure 1. The Bell Curve Model of Health and Medicine

The reference point for this statistical analysis and determination of what is considered to be healthy is based on the study of a large group of individuals, most often white men.

Individuals whose health results fall outside the statistical norms are deemed abnormal and/or diseased. This bell curve model of health implies that the most frequently occurring conditions in a human population define an impartial, scientific notion of health and normality. Additionally, in the bell curve model, diseases are universal. Given the same biological circumstances and causes, individuals all over the world will develop the same disorders. Time, place, environment, and social arrangements have very little to no role in the incidence of disease.

The *bell curve model of health* is how mainstream medicine sees health. This is synonymous with *small health*. *Bell curve medicine* is the way mainstream medicine treats patients according to bell curve statistical norms. This is synonymous with *small medicine*.

In the bell curve model of health, disease is an outlier experience separated from the statistical range of health. Inside the bell curve are the normative experiences considered synonymous with health. In this model, health is also linked to additional normative processes around age, weight, body shape, physical activity, mood, and thinking. This means that good health depends upon how old you are, how much you weigh, how active your lifestyle is, and how even-tempered and balanced your mood is. If you are beyond a certain age or above a certain body weight, you will experience being automatically excluded from the bell curve model of health.

The bell curve view of normality and health is so pervasive that it has hypnotized an entire society into thinking in its terms. This social construction of health dominates our thinking and influences how we treat outlier experiences.

The Croatian-Austrian philosopher Ivan Illich once said, "The pursuit of health may be a sickening disorder."[8] Like Illich, I postulate that we need to reduce our concerns with health. In *Health in Sickness, Sickness in Health,* I argued that our current social interpretation of health adds a layer of sickness to the illness experience of many people. The centrality of health puts pressure on us when we are healthy as well as when we are sick. For example, when we feel the onset of a cold, with a sore throat, low energy, and a clouded mind, most of us will respond by taking vitamins and herbs to fight the virus while continuing on with our regular activities. In so doing, we miss out on the opportunity to let ourselves slow down and take care of our need to turn inward. The pressure to be extroverted and to fit goes against our more diverse needs that sometimes direct us to take a time out.

Bell curve medicine is about fighting disease to get back under the roof of normality and all its privileges. Big Medicine is about using medical knowledge and techniques to treat the disease while also engaging in the art of living life with all its diverse experiences, some of which don't fall under the curve. I posit that the outlier experiences have the chance to enrich our lives by bringing awareness to diverse aspects of ourselves and our communities.

As stated above, health is only one of many normative processes that are imposed on society. The bell curve model of health overlaps and interacts with other social norms based on communication style, behavior, class, culture, skin color, gender, size, and sexual orientation.

If you are a woman of color living in poverty, your chance of fitting within the bell curve of health correlates with your exposure to racism and sexism. Systemic oppression from these and other factors, as well as exposure to trauma and adverse childhood events, are insults to individuals' physical and emotional integrity and affect our ability to fit within health norms.

Here is an example of this complex intersectionality—specifically between class, trauma, and health. Some time ago, I participated in a care conference for a client of mine. Alex is a middle-aged, single father who suffers from severe and disabling Crohn's disease, an autoimmune inflammation of the bowels. Over the years, Alex has undergone several surgeries with many ensuing complications, including the need to have a colostomy, an artificial opening of his intestines. Carrying a pouch in which his feces would drain made him feel embarrassment and shame. It interfered with his ability to have meaningful relationships at work and in his personal life.

In his youth and early adulthood, Alex experienced multiple traumas. As a poor white male, he was jailed at an early age for drug-related offenses, and the mother of his child committed suicide. The chronic physical pain from his Crohn's and the chronic emotional and psychological pain from his life experiences made him an angry and short-tempered man. This affected his relationship with his teenage son, and in an attempt to improve this relationship, Alex self-medicated his anger with marijuana, which helped but also often caused nausea and vomiting.

Alex's medical providers frequently complained about his combative stances towards them and his lack of compliance with their treatment recommendations. Nonetheless, Alex fought for a restorative surgical procedure to get rid of his colostomy. With difficulty, he eventually found a surgeon who agreed to perform this risky surgery.

The surgery initially went well. But for some unknown reason, Alex left the hospital against medical recommendation. Once at home, he smoked a joint that made him vomit. This put too much pressure on the surgical wound and led the scars to burst open. It created a huge fistula with a new abdominal opening of his gut. Alex was back at square one, only now with an even worse stoma. This time, to allow for wound healing, he was asked to stop ingesting any food or fluid and was put on total parenteral nutrition (TPN), nutrition that is directly infused into the blood circulation. Alex was not able to comply with this mandate to not eat or drink, which led to a standoff with his medical care team and to the care conference I participated in. His trauma and disease, and the systemic oppression he experienced because of his class and upbringing, ultimately led Alex to die an early death.

Social Pressure to Be Healthy

The push toward health and healing—or moving toward the inside of the bell curve—is, because of its conformist aspect, psychologically and emotionally oppressive. As such, it elicits resistance. This is one reason why patients' compliance with medical recommendations hovers around 50 percent.[9] The pressure to fit in and be healthy conflicts with their unconscious wish to be allowed to be different. This dynamic is most significant for people with chronic conditions and disabilities.

Fitting within the curve is a privilege that is not attainable to all; for some, it's not even something they want to aim for. The mainstream medical model devalues the outlier experience and denies its rightful existence, as well as the identity and culture that comes with it.

The majority culture's process of mainstreaming[10] our health has oppressive overtones that we could call "healthist" (similar to "sexist" or "racist") because mainstreaming disregards the meaning of the illness experience and the peer identity that can come with it. In medical school, I was trained to explore, when confronted with non-compliant patients, the "secondary gain" or benefit they might draw from their illness. This was deemed to be a psychological or emotional problem that interfered with treatment and healing. For example, we assumed that non-compliant patients were seeking attention through their illness, and we were taught to help them develop more appropriate and healthy ways of gaining attention. I rather think we need to add a new perspective that accepts the possibility of true value in aspects of illness and disease experiences.

The bell curve model of health pathologizes not only the physiological disease process and the mechanics of our bodies' malfunctions but also the illness experience — the subjective experiences that accompany disease. Individuals who experience a process outside of the health norm are cast out from the rest of the allegedly healthy society and use the same standards to blame themselves for this as well.

This societal norming happens in the fields of both physical and mental health. Some disorders come with a greater social stigma than others. AIDS is a good example of a highly stigmatized physical disease. In behavioral health, illicit substance abuse and delusional, psychotic, or anger-related behaviors are prone to more intense marginalization. Those individuals with such processes often internalize the outer stigma and the notion of pathology and use it against themselves. A whole range of experiences are medicalized and judged against a norm of health, both externally in society's perception and internally, in one's own self-evaluation.

An ancient Greek myth illustrates the dynamics of these social demands. Procrustes, the mythic ogre, was an innkeeper along the road to Athens, the metropolis of Greek culture. Voyagers on their journey to Athens spent their last night in Procrustes's inn. While they were asleep, Procrustes retrofitted the travelers' bodies to his one-size iron bed by cutting down or stretching their limbs.

As a guard of Greek social conventions and rules, Procrustes re-aligned his guests to the mainstream culture's norms. By adopting the bell curve model of health, we all act like Procrustes. We marginalize the outlier experience to fit within health norm. We pathologize our own illness experiences, hoping to be accepted by our culture and community.

Illness and Addiction Processes and Big Medicine

Big Medicine sees disease and illness as a Process—an aspect of the ever-evolving nature of life, with its endless diversity of experiences. Process with a capital "P" stands for the inherent tendency of life's manifestations to be dynamic, multi-layered, and forward moving. Every experience is constantly changing and in flow. Some experiences benefit from medical interventions, but they are not wrong, bad, or abnormal. On the contrary, even the most painful experience has the potential to bring us more awareness.

Big Medicine avoids identifying individuals and groups with their disease or illness. It doesn't use terms like "addicts," "depressed people," or "diabetics." People have a Process; they are not the condition they suffer from. We are people who have Processes, conditions, and experiences—some "good" and some "bad." We are individuals who experience life with all its natural occurrences.

A person with a substance use or diabetes Process needs support to navigate, cope with, and hopefully recover from what afflicts them. Untying their identity from the disease minimizes the stigma and shame that comes with the illness and allows them to explore that Process with curiosity.

For example, a client I am coaching is fighting an addiction to marijuana. He tells me that he often smokes when he feels bored, and that when he smokes, his thoughts and feelings are more intense and vibrant. He becomes more excited about his own inner creative process. In my work with him, I explored his barriers toward being passionate and excited about his creativity. Together, we looked at ways he can counter his inner critic, who stifles his attempts to write poetry. We discovered that his boredom often arises when he fails to believe in his creative projects. Nonetheless, the creative unfolding of his Process doesn't exclude his need to quit smoking marijuana.

Just the other day, I explored with my client Kristen her long-term experience of struggling with depression and the lingering fear of getting depressed again. Her depression came with a feeling of being constrained and very internal. She likened the depression to an ice-cold power that would pull her down and inward. She associated that power with the cold piercing blue eyes of the Night King from the TV show *Game of Thrones*.

When I suggested she deepen her experience, Kristen imagined the characteristics of the Night King's kingdom as well as sounds or music that would emanate from his world. She expressed them in movement and with her voice, falling into a dance with sounds that reminded her of ringing ice crystals and reverberating Balinese bells. This exercise helped her get in touch with an internal, "cold," or detached musical strength that she possesses but is shy about.

Asked if she could imagine herself somehow bringing this power into life, she expressed the urge to be more outwardly engaged in a world that needed her political advocacy. She felt she wasn't suited for political action because she imagined it would require her to be more extroverted and passionate, which didn't fit her personality. Not knowing how to be an introverted activist, she became hopeless.

Our work together then evolved into ways of using her intuitive, clairvoyant, and crystalline intelligence in everyday life and political action. Is there a causal link between her struggle to be actively engaged in her community and her depression? Or was she depressed because she wasn't acknowledging her desire to be politically active? Whatever the sequence of cause and effect, unfolding the experience creatively shed light on her internal conflict; it put her depression in a meaningful context of competing motivations.

The medical model sees depression as a condition that falls outside the normal distribution of human functioning. It's a deviation from the average physiological workings of the majority of the population. Because of genetic dispositions and environmental factors, the depressed person's brain chemistry becomes abnormal, out of the standard range of how neurotransmitters normally work. This creates the sufferer's symptoms of low energy, lack of pleasure, and depressed mood. Treatment logically focuses on the restoration of normal brain chemistry and functioning.

Big Medicine, in contrast, uses a different definition of health, one that integrates the outlier or deviant illness experience. It sees depression as not only a pathological condition. The distressing symptoms give, if supported by a wondering and inquisitive attitude, access to a new world with its own wisdom and intelligence. In this approach, nobody is deemed abnormal or unhealthy. Instead, people have various "Dreaming" experiences that bring them into contact with unlived or marginalized aspects of their Process (Process Work uses the term *Dreaming* to emphasize the dreamlike quality of our subjective illness experiences. These experiences are doors into a poetic dream world, which, when unfolded, give us access to valuable information). Biomedical interventions are important, but they are not the whole story. They can make us miss the opportunity to explore the potential purpose and meaning of our own or our client's holistic Process. That Process, as we will see, encompasses multiple levels of experiences, only one of which is the bell curve model of health.

In a counseling practice, it is very common to see severely traumatized clients who engage in behaviors and take in substances that alter their mind. They are often very self-critical, putting themselves down for all sorts of things as well as their addiction. If, as a counselor, you side with the critic by pathologizing their behavior, you tend to reinforce the cycle of trauma and victimization. By using a Big Medicine approach, you might be able to help the client recognize their true Dreaming and shamanic nature, which is the best medicine you can offer to help them overcome their trauma history.

A colleague of mine worked with a client whose family history included abusive relationships and suicide. He was bullied in school, and at a young age he was institutionalized for fear he would avenge himself with violence. His ongoing mandated treatment reinforced his self-doubt and insecurities. In a recent dream, he visited his abusive ancestor's ranch and noticed that the pasture around the ranch was beautifully green.

My colleague remarked on the thriving green surroundings of the dream ranch and helped her client let go of the family trauma and focus on his own thriving and achievements. Rather than perpetuating the abuse by centering on it, she shifted the focus to what was healthy in her client's experience. As counselors and healthcare providers, we tend to equate trauma with damage and by focusing on the trauma freeze our clients into an identity of feeling victimized. A Big Medicine attitude allows us to appreciate the entirety of the client's process, facilitate its unfolding, and foster resilience.

Conventional medical science aggregates health and body stories and categorizes them into separate groups. In so doing, it identifies patterns that have better outcomes in terms of reduced impairment and longer lives. Big Medicine, in contrast, looks at individual stories and processes. It explores the foreign languages and landscapes of body symptoms as a means to discovering a new world full of information and meaning, both for the individual and his or her community.

Within the bell curve model of health, the starting point is the pathology, the objectively abnormal biology of the disease process. The subjective and social illness experiences are byproducts of the material dysfunction. If the body machine malfunctions, it creates secondary side effects that are of lesser importance. The subjective symptoms are relevant only as signposts for the discovery of the disease that needs to be eradicated. As mentioned earlier, in this machine-like medical model, diseases are universal and invariant to time, place, the individual experiencing the disease, and his or her social environment.

Illness, Quantum Physics, and the Nature of Reality

Bell curve medicine continues to perceive reality in classical physical or Newtonian terms, where everything is determined in space and time. The real world is like the body of a machine governed by the laws of classical physics, such as gravity, motion, and temperature.

In contrast, the fundamental laws of quantum physics (e.g., wave-particle duality and quantum entanglement) are probabilistic, forcing us to abandon the notion of precisely defined causal and linear trajectories, such as A causes B. We cannot tell anymore what, how, or where something is. The mathematical equations of quantum physics give us only approximations. At the subatomic level, the laws of physics become more ambiguous, nebulous, and dreamlike.

Our current definitions of health and disease are shaped by Newtonian classical physics. In this world, health and disease, life and death, exclude each other; they can't exist simultaneously. From a quantum perspective, these identifiable and differentiated states are not opposites—and they are also not the whole story. There is a deeper reality of potentialities, a world where something can be both a particle and a wave, and where observation is required even to manifest the particle or wave nature.

Recall my client with cervical cancer. In our work together, we fluctuated between addressing the particle and wave aspects of her cancer. Initially, she was focused on the difficulty of choosing the right course of treatment: How to decide between surgery and/or radiation therapy; how to estimate and balance the risks and benefits. This attended to the more particle-like nature of the cancer and its treatment. Later, we explored the more dream- or wave-like aspects of her subjective experience: Her fears and imagination about how it might impact her sexuality and what it would mean to possibly become incontinent.

During one session, I helped her get into the mindset of a cancer cell and explore what it was about. I offered her a basket full of toys and puppets from which to choose something that could represent that malignant cell. She immediately pulled out a black puppet that was part spider and part bat. I didn't remember having this puppet, but she had a strong emotional reaction to it. A playful interaction ensued, in which we explored ways of behaving more like a bat or a spider, relying on ultrasonic senses and a web of filaments, being more intrusive and invasive in the way she imagined a cancer cell would behave but with ultrasound-like sensitivity and the delicateness of a spider web.

Living in modern society, we are hyper-attuned to the particle aspects of disease, but we need some encouragement to delve into the dreamlike wave realm. The Dreaming happens to us in irrational intuitions and fantasies, in night dreams about our disease Process, and in synchronicities and serendipitous events around the disease Process.

If we return to the bell curve graph and look at it with a quantum perspective, health and illness are manifested actualities that emerge from a unified field of potential states or experiences. Is there a meaning to this diversity of experiences? Why does this differentiating process out of a pluripotent realm occur? One theory is that differentiation allows for the emergence of consciousness. In the soup of potentialities without differentiation, there is no awareness; awareness requires contrast or distinction. Without disease, we would not know what health is. Without her cervical cancer, my client would not have had the opportunity to bolster her ultrasonic sensibility and invasive nature. Disease is an expression of reality that is needed to create diversity, and through diversity, more awareness.

And then, as we will explore more in detail later in this book, reality does not just exist out there in the world waiting to be discovered. It is co-created by individuals and societies in a process of consensus building. Our understanding of reality and the world is shaped by our current social arrangements and cultural conventions and norms. As our knowledge and social world change over time, so do our perceptions of reality.

Identity and Health/Illness

Every day, we have a multitude of experiences, some of which are more familiar and comfortable than others. It makes sense to align our more comfortable experiences with a preferred notion, such as health, and to relegate the other more uncomfortable ones to the domain of illness. But deep down, they come from the same unified field, and their separation helps us become more aware. The meanings we assign to them are shaped by common sense, social arrangements, and cultural norms. From an evolutionary viewpoint, the preferable health state gives the individual and communities a greater advantage. So, again, it makes sense that we prioritize health over illness.

This is especially relevant when it comes to so-called "chronic" health conditions and disabilities, experiences around which individuals develop peer identities.[11] It explains why new healing technologies and treatments (such as cochlear implants) are confronted with resistance from some. For many, being deaf is considered a disability. But for others, especially for individuals who were born without the ability to hear, this condition is just another type of existence. They are members of a different culture without sound perception, one in which being Deaf is normal. Reversing deafness through medical interventions becomes a negation of cultural identity and disability rights. Health, normality—in this instance, hearing—becomes a critique of a diverse lifestyle and culture. For them, the peer Deaf culture is one to be proud and not ashamed of.

When our physician, using the bell curve model, diagnoses us with an illness, he or she changes our behavior. We feel we are no longer whole and we need to fight to return to the land of health. Obviously, health is a preferred state, and every sensible human being will try to recover as quickly as possible. In collaboration with our physician, we decide the best course of action to get back under the bell curve of health. Together, as patients and providers, we determine the standards for health and normality, including which conditions we accept as legitimate illnesses, which ones we delegitimize or stigmatize, and which ones we claim for access to disability benefits. In so doing, we are adding a social state to our biophysiological state. Procrustes, the enforcer of social norms, is very alive in all of us.

The Big Medicine lens, in addition to embracing the aspects of bell curve medicine that make sense, opens to a wider angle. It sees health and illness as one burgeoning tree rooted in the earth, with multiple intertwined branches expressing differentiation and awareness. Both health and illness are opportunities for discovery and learning. One culture is more familiar and prioritized—that of health. The other, illness or disease, is more foreign and marginal. The amount of time we are granted to spend in the land of health depends on serendipity, luck, privilege, genes, and individual choices and behaviors. Sooner or later, we all must travel through illness territory.

Because health is our comfort zone, it keeps us unconscious. Illness and disease, in contrast, force us to wake up. Learning the dream- or wave-like language and symbols of our subjective illness experiences gives us access to greater awareness and knowledge of the deeper nature of reality at its universal and timeless level. For my client with cervical cancer, unfolding the symbols of her cancer cell metaphors gave her some insight into unknown parts of herself. At a later stage, our work might evolve into helping her embrace her own diversity and connect with her own roots and branches that express all the various experiences.

When illness throws us into this foreign landscape and culture, everything in us wants to escape. Recall my client who suffered consecutive brain injuries from two car accidents. No one would blame her if her only pursuit were recovery and returning to the familiar landscape of health. The fact that she was open to learning a new language of illness is extraordinary.

Health Refugees

⌣

A friend told me a harrowing story that relates to this discussion. One evening, my friend's wife and her sister went to a restaurant and ate fish and chips. That night, the sister felt that something was really wrong; she experienced weird numbness in her face and feared she was dying. An ER visit didn't help elucidate what was happening to her, and the symptoms slowly faded away. Months later, the sister was visiting with some friends and ate fish. This time, she became violently ill. A nurse herself, she thought she had food poisoning again and coped with the disease.

But from that night on, she started experiencing both gastrointestinal and neurological symptoms. She could not keep much food down, and the numbness and tingling around her mouth came back. It took many doctor visits for her before she learned she had Ciguatera fish poisoning, in which a toxin enters and stays inside human cells and becomes active when triggered by the consumption of certain foods. There is no remedy. Affected individuals recover slowly, or symptoms can persist and lead to disability. My friend's wife had also eaten fish and chips, but she must not have eaten a contaminated piece. One sister was lucky; the other was struck by a fateful event that may well change her whole life.

In my day job, I work with political and religious refugees who have been forced out of their homeland. This is what happens to people who experience such fateful diseases and accidents: They are suddenly expelled from the land of the healthy into the no-man's-land of chronic illness. To expect them to be open to considering learning a new language and finding meaning in their experience is almost impossible. Their main experience is one of powerlessness and of being traumatized by what is happening to them. Any refugee, if they had a choice, would want to return to their homeland and prior life. Health refugees are no different.

So, what can a Big Medicine approach bring? First, it acknowledges that mainstream thinking delineates borders between health-land and illness-land and that patients deserve refugee status. The medically determined standards of normality and health create boundaries that exclude us when we are ill. This happens to all of us, but some of us are alienated at an earlier age and for longer time periods. The boundaries keep the unlucky ones out and prevent them from getting back in. Keeping these rigid standards is like building high concrete walls that protect the healthy and keep others out of the country of health.

Then, Big Medicine helps individuals and communities learn the new languages and cultures of their subjective illness and impairment experiences. It helps them adjust to their refugee status and learn the language and culture of the new host country. It also helps us all loosen our rigid boundaries around the meaning of "health," so we can integrate other diverse experiences into a more unified country.

Big Medicine facilitates the communication between health refugees and health-typical individuals. By giving a voice to illness and disease, it brings awareness to health as a diversity problem and social justice issue. There is no health here and disease there. There is only health diversity, disease diversity, and illness diversity.

Bell curve medicine creates a hierarchy and ranking of experiences, assigning more access to resources and privileges to those who are more fortunate and healthy. Big Medicine sheds light on the intersection of health and social disparities, expands our knowledge of ourselves and our peers, and tears down the wall that separates illness-land from health-land. We all experience health, disease, illness, and ultimately death. We all have very diverse experiences of these, and we can learn from each other and help minimize the marginalization of ill health.

Whereas ease and comfort lull us into sleepwalking and inertia, it's life's disruptors that wake us up. Big Medicine, with its attention to the language and meaning of disease, brings us closer to fundamental existential questions such as, What am I? What am I here for? Why am I suffering? What does my illness mean? Paradoxically, by integrating the disavowed language and culture of disease, Big Medicine fosters a deeper understanding of the purpose and meaning of life.

Meghan O'Rourke writes in *The New Yorker*[12] about her experience with chronic autoimmune disease:

> What I had wasn't just an illness now; it was an identity, a membership in a peculiarly demanding sect. I had joined the First Assembly of the Diffusely Unwell. The Church of Fatigue, Itching, and Random Neuralgia. Temple Beth Ill.

Her piece powerfully describes her journey into the no-man's-land of chronic illness, her expulsion from her old identity, and her struggles to cope and survive. She quotes the French writer Alphonse Daudet from *In the Land of Pain*: "Pain is always new to the sufferer, but loses its originality for those around him."

This is the divide that severely and chronically ill people experience—a divide that is maintained by those of us who hide behind the wall of so-called "good health" and bell curve medicine. "Healthy" people stop wanting to hear about the suffering. O'Rourke describes her need to find peer sufferers: a community of individuals who speak the same language and understand each other's change of cultural health identity.

Peers can, over time and despite feeling marginalized, develop a sense of pride and positive identity that embraces their health diversity. Today, peer support services are gaining much-deserved attention in addiction recovery, mental health, and other health subcultures. They can help people with illness experiences find community, regain some power, and balance the healthism of dominant culture.

Putting New Perspectives into Practice

If you would like to practice applying Big Medicine approaches to your own physical symptom or illness experiences, try the following inner work exercises.

Inner work is a practice of becoming involved with your inner experiences that can lead to a transformation of your sense of self. It can encompass, for instance, meditation, religious practices, and Process-informed psychological work. When we practice inner work, we notice an inner experience, review the event that led to the experience, and reflect on our own actions and the actions of others. We also examine the feelings, memories, sensations, and images that are associated with the event or the experience itself. Inner work allows us to identify our conditioned and socialized responses and discover new options.[13]

Take a moment to feel your body and choose one experience it is having. Keep your focus on this experience, noticing any physical sensations as well as associated memories and images. For example, my head feels slightly heavy and altered. I am remembering last night's party and friends' comments that made me feel self-critical. The echoes of the self-defeating thoughts contribute to my altered state, and when I stay with this experience, I go silent and internal and find a peaceful, more detached place within myself.

If you find yourself feeling self-critical about an aspect of your health, such as a perceived addiction, you can try approaching it from a Big Medicine viewpoint instead of a bell curve medicine perspective. Imagine using the substance or engaging in the behavior and recall how this feels in your body and mind. Does it create a certain physical feeling, emotion, or altered state? Look at yourself from inside that experience, exploring the illness culture created by that altered state. Deliberate with your inner critic and facilitate a dialogue between your conventional self, your altered self, and the critic.

You can also use the more detailed steps in the next exercise to understand the deeper meaning of one of your physical symptoms.

Inner Work Exercise: Illness Narrative

1. Choose a physical symptom or illness you are currently experiencing.

2. Look at it from inside the bell curve, the conventional viewpoint that sees this symptom or illness as a disease that needs to be cured. What are your thoughts and insights from this vantage point?

3. Step into the experience of the symptom. Notice the body part it is in, take time to feel it, its specific qualities; is it hot, cold, sharp, dull, pounding, or burning? Amplify the experience by allowing it to expand, by breathing into that symptom area, or by drawing an image of it or making a sound that captures its quality.

4. Turn the symptom experience into a metaphorical figure who embodies the illness language and culture. Imagine what kind of a human-like figure would embody the quality of your symptom. For example, if you experience a pounding headache, what kind of a powerful figure would embody the pounding?

5. Step into the role of Procrustes, the innkeeper who makes everyone fit the same bed, and ask yourself, What is wrong in identifying with the figure who impersonates the symptom experience?

6. Look at yourself from the vantage point of the illness figure.

7. Create a dialogue between you, the bell curve perspective, and the illness figure.

To help you get started, I will share an example from my own life. I suffer from allergic nasal irritation and inflammation that lead to itching, sneezing, a runny nose, and nasal congestion. From inside the bell curve, this experience irritates me. I want to get rid of it, so I use a nasal spray.

But if I allow myself to run with the symptom experience, I let the nose drool and sneeze and express all its reactions to environmental triggers. I become a very sensitive and expressive person who shares all his feelings and reactions. The figure I associate with such behavior is one of a court jester or fool, who speaks his mind and doesn't follow customary communication protocols. As Procrustes, I curtail my spontaneity and expression of my feelings to fit in and not upset the conventions. As the jester, I pick up and express all the environmental and atmospheric tensions to clear the air.

I grew up in a family environment in which feelings were considered private and kept away from the dinner table and other conversations. This family culture originates in a Calvinistic Protestant tradition. My maternal grandfather was an accomplished Swiss diplomat who was stern in his demeanor and who never cussed. His strongest expression of dissatisfaction was "nom d'une pipe," which translates as "for goodness' sake." In his culture, it was considered a sacrilege to cuss and specially to use the name of God in swear words. This stance seeped through his every interaction, and besides its good intent of maintaining polite communication, it also oppressed strong feelings.

That debate or culture war is ongoing in my allergic rhinitis. This relatively harmless but annoying symptom irritates me. It irritates my sense of comfort and well-being—and, on a deeper level, my identity as someone who avoids rocking the boat in relationships. A Big Medicine approach gives me more awareness and choices for how to transgress my identity boundaries and develop a new relationship culture in which I can express all my feelings. It also allows me to experience my illness in a different way and stop relegating it to a refugee status.

Chapter 3

BIG HEALTH AND BIG MEDICINE

L ET'S RETURN TO the doctor's office. But now, imagine that you're in the office of a future practitioner of Big Medicine. You are sitting comfortably in a welcoming and trauma-informed environment. Before performing any tests, the doctor listened to your story with curiosity. She is excited to help you understand what is going on and what your body is telling you. She shares her own fallibility and questions as she processes the test results with you. (For more details about self-disclosure, see the section "Big Medicine for Patients and Providers" in Chapter 6.) She explains that test results are not the whole story and that your personal experience is more relevant than any test. She helps you delve more deeply into your embodied experience, so you can develop a relationship with this unfamiliar set of symptoms. She treats you with respect and interest in your wholeness.

Because Big Health is such a radical new way of conceptualizing health, I will reiterate its basic tenets. In Big Health, health becomes a Process that includes the experiences of feeling sick and disabled. In addition to avoiding, preventing, and combating disease, it welcomes the outlier experiences as an expression of diversity and as an exciting opportunity for expanding our knowledge and identities. Big Health embraces the smooth and warm sandy beaches of our existence, as well as the sharp, icy, windy, and rocky mountains. Together, health and sickness are expressions of the most fundamental Process: your meaningful passage through life.

Big Medicine uses the concepts of process-oriented psychology and Big Health to carve out a path for healing and personal growth. It gives us a new medicine cabinet for self-healing. Big Medicine revisits and deepens the concepts of Big Health with a lens on how to make it applicable for Process-informed growth and healing. The path of Big Medicine begins with the key subjective experiences of individual and community ill health. Big Medicine then gives us a compass and traveler's guidebook to navigate the various geographies and weather patterns of health and illness.

There is ample critique of what I call the bell curve model of health. Aaron Antonovsky, Ivan Illich, Thomas Szasz, Susan Sontag, R.D. Laing, Larry Dossey, and David Cooper are some of the many scholars who have challenged mainstream approaches to health, disease, and the concept and relevance of diagnoses in both medicine and psychiatry.

But it is the German philosopher Friedrich Nietzsche who questioned the very idea of "health" as such. He objected to the notion of a "normal" health and of generalizable therapeutic procedures.

In *The Gay Science,* Nietzsche[14] writes:

> A health per se does not exist.... It depends on your goal, your horizon, your powers, your drive, your mistakes, and in particular, on the ideals and phantasms of your soul in order to determine what health even means for your body.... Last, the big question is still open if we could dispense with disease ... if the sole desire for health is not a prejudice, a cowardice, and perhaps a piece of finest barbarism and backwardness.

To this he contrasts a *grosse Gesundheit,* a Big Health that is always a process, never static and never to be fully achieved and attained. One can never *have* health, as we always lose it and need to find it again.

He compares our quest for health to a hero's journey in search for an ideal.

Nietzsche himself suffered from many chronic health problems. He struggled with debilitating migraine headaches, near-sightedness, abdominal cramps, and environmental sensitivities, as well as paralysis and speech problems. In later years, he experienced mental breakdowns. He saw health and illness as processes in the context of one's existential path and purpose. He concluded that illnesses are necessary obstacles on the path toward health; they can be motivating experiences and allies in a new creative process.

Big Health is like the quest of Jason and his Argonauts, who sailed the oceans of ancient Greece to find the Golden Fleece. Health is a utopian ideal, never to be fully reached, a journey fraught with dangers and challenges. This is in stark contrast to a naturalistic view of health, in which the human body and its organs have objective normal functions, and diseases are aberrations of this ideal functioning.

Big Health as a hero's quest—a developmental process in search of a utopian ideal—stands in opposition to a bell curve model of health in which the ideal is a statistical norm that we deviate from as we get sick and age.

A few weeks ago, I consulted with a woman who was fighting a recurrence of breast cancer. Despite feeling sick she still had many reasons to live and projects to complete, she feared death was looming around the corner. In our work, she was able to face death as it was sneaking in, reminding her to be attentive to the sound of the birds and the warmth of the sunlight. We happened to be in Israel at an international conference, where we were surrounded by groves of citrus trees. I helped her identify with the essence of the orange trees and their particular scent. She embodied a tree and expressed its expansive and vibrant energy as well as its warmth. In unfolding her experience, death became an ally that helped her rediscover a forgotten quality of her own nature.

From a small health perspective, breast cancer is a biological malfunction that throws the afflicted off the path of health (and for some, ultimately, life). Bell curve health is like a means of transportation along the meandering road of life. Diseases are roadblocks, boulders, potholes, and other obstacles that challenge our forward movement. Some people are given a truck, motorbike, bicycle, four-wheel drive, or luxury automobile to tackle the journey, while others have the privilege of traveling less hazardous roads.

In contrast, in Big Health, health is the whole journey. It is not only the mechanical vehicle that carries us, but the entirety of the expedition and discovery. Diseases are intrinsic features of the landscape along the way. Breast cancer and the fear of death transform from being threats into reminders of our own intrinsic participation in the panorama of nature and life.

In a bell curve world, we travel through life as tourists hoping to encounter the fewest obstacles possible and to travel outside of the most foreign and dangerous terrain. Injuries, insults, and malfunctions are distractions and challenges, and we seek the help of mechanics to regain free and undisturbed passage. We bypass other less fortunate tourists who are stranded, looking away to avoid being reminded of our own risks along the journey.

In a bell curve paradigm, we marginalize illness and the ill. But in a Big Health paradigm, we all inhabit the same world and participate in its creation. Death, diseases, injuries, and disabilities are specific characteristics of the natural world we are all discovering together. From this perspective, my client was not only suffering from breast cancer and the fear of possibly immanent death—but rediscovering that she was the orange tree with its enchanting, warm, and vibrant scent.

We want the mechanics of bell curve health to help us identify and treat our bodies' malfunctions, but our quest for Big Health and meaning does not depend on health. The bell curve model of health and its glitches are rooted in the body and its physiological mechanisms. Big Health hinges on the body and its functioning but is not determined by it.

For example, it's impossible to understand Big Health in terms of classical Newtonian mechanics and chemistry. Big Health requires the addition of quantum physics and relativity. Arnold Mindell reminds us that, although Einstein's Theory of Relativity describes how large masses bend the space-time continuum and create gravitational pulls, the speed of light is not affected and remains constant across all universes.[15] Physical and emotional challenges can act as large masses that drag us down, but the light of awareness remains accessible and free. Mind and awareness, although rooted in our bodies, remain available even when our bodies are extremely impaired, such as in comatose or near-death states.[16]

Big Health, as an achievable state, is a fiction — it doesn't exist, just as diseases and pathologies do not exist in its world. Big Health is an attitude and mindset. It is awareness of the process-oriented properties of Nature.

The mechanics of bell curve health can be taught, and doctors and other health professionals can learn which medicine can fix the small health disruptions. Big Health, however, cannot be taught. We can be inspired and mentored to step out of the bell curve health world, to get out of our cars and discover Nature and Process. Once outside the car, outside of bell curve health, we can learn to appreciate the diversity of our experiences.

Recall the woman from Chapter 2 who was poisoned by Ciguatera. Struggling with her illness, she has lost weight and her appearance has changed dramatically. Her friends comment to each other about how sick and frail she looks and how fast her hair is going gray. To her face, they are caring and offer their advice. The friends are, like many of us, hypnotized by bell curve health, which views illness as pathology and flavors it with lookism, ageism, and sexism.

My client with breast cancer, too, receives more well-intentioned concern and health advice than is helpful to her. Her friends' comments convey their expectation of her poor small health prognosis and implied death sentence. Small health holds all of us hostage to a reductionist worldview and concept of health. This adds a layer of unnecessary social and psychological harm to what is already a most challenging experience—coping with a serious illness. The bell curve health bias has a *nocebo* effect, a detrimental psychological impact that comes with negative expectations and mindsets. It certainly depresses people and at times even kills them.

The Big Health attitude values the knowledge and tools of bell curve health and medicine. But it doesn't allow them to dominate the whole range of experiences. Awareness, learning, and growth are the constants, and they are always freely accessible. We may be sick, traumatized, in pain, and caught up in messy relationships. These are as great an opportunity to learn and grow as when we feel well and happy. In fact, good health and emotional well-being can actually make us too comfortable and lazy.

Pathology

Pathology is the causal study of diseases, their material etiology (or origin), and the clinical manifestations, symptoms, and illnesses they produce. Diagnoses are decisions that medical professionals reach based on the signs and symptoms that patients experience; they are synonymous with the names of the diseases. They enable health professionals to develop a common understanding and language. Pathology and diagnoses stand in contrast to the normal and healthy functioning of the body. Over the past century, the concept of pathology has expanded into the realm of behaviors and thought, thus extending the medical model into psychiatry, psychology, and other social sciences.

Many diagnoses are subject to moral judgment and stigmatization, such as HIV and other sexually transmitted diseases. Obesity is another; individuals who suffer weight-related health problems are often chastised for overeating or being too sedentary. Any form of addiction is blamed on the individual. Very few health professionals are aware of the social determinants of health and the responsibility of a vast array of industries that actively promote addictive behaviors to increase their revenue.

Besides objective physiological norms, we now have psychological, behavioral, and cognitive norms and standards. Pathology has infected the way we think about our bodies, health, relationships, behaviors, community interactions, mental processes, and internalized views of ourselves. Normative thinking—designating some experiences as pathological (disease) and others as normal (health)—has become a pervasive mode of judging. As medical thinking expands into psychological and social spheres, medical value-based judgments of health and sickness are infusing every sphere of our lives. Small health has become the standard lens through which we view both the outside world and our inner worlds.

The concept of pathology relies on a dual way of thinking, or Boolean logic. A person is either healthy or sick, dead or alive; it is either 1 or 0. This duality creates contrast and differentiation. It helps us identify a dysfunction, name it with a diagnosis, and then suggest treatment options in hopes of reversing it.

Many of the refugees whom I work with have survived horrendous experiences. Because I work in a clinical environment that requires me to justify the use of government funds, I have to come up with a recognized medical diagnosis that then establishes the medical necessity of my services. The refugees' most frequent clinical presentation is one of post-traumatic stress, the diagnosis being post-traumatic stress disorder, or PTSD. From a social justice lens, PTSD is a normal reaction to abnormal circumstances, making it hard to call it a "disease." War, ethnic cleansing, and other political traumas produce psychological and social injuries. To treat them as individual pathologies ignores the political causes and adds another layer of injustice.

Other forms of oppression and abuse—such as domestic violence, racism, sexism, and homophobia—are even more pervasive than war and ethnic-based conflicts. All have damaging health effects, and all have their roots in societal factors. To treat them as if they are individual problems is to blame the victim. The Kaiser Permanente Adverse

Childhood Experiences Study[17] and other research papers that demonstrate the deleterious effect of trauma, abuse, inequality, and social marginalization highlight the importance of community-inflicted trauma in creating pathology and sickness. Suddenly, what causes pathology becomes more complicated and multidimensional. At the intersection of individual lives and community, the development of a malignant cell that will grow into a cancerous tumor—a pathology that is clearly demarcated—is now a complex process that depends on multiple overlapping factors.

Recently, two of my colleagues worked with a woman who was suffering from what she, as a health practitioner, called "irritable bowel syndrome with constipation," or IBS-C, a condition that had started in her teenage years 20 years before. No medical or dietary treatment had helped. She experienced the chronic constipation as bloating, a sense of abdominal pressure, fullness, and "stuckness."

In their session, one of my colleagues asked her to physically recreate the symptoms in him. She started pushing and applying pressure to his belly. In the process, she realized it was not she who was doing this, but that she had somehow become her father pressuring her. With a great deal of emotion, she recalled his abusive behavior toward her during the time when her symptoms started.

My colleagues then helped her respond to the pressure by pushing back. Initially, she was very hesitant, saying this was not how she would want to act. This made a lot of sense, as she didn't want to be like her father who had hurt her so badly. With some encouragement, she stepped into a playful physical interaction, finally forcefully pushing one of my colleagues against the wall and expressing her resolve and anger.

As a group, we discussed the social sanctions against women showing and embodying their power and anger and how all of us censor ourselves for reasons that relate to society and our personal history.

That same afternoon, I had worked with a woman who was suffering from persistent depression. She was struggling with wanting to continue to live in a world that she perceived as murderous. She had experienced the traumatic loss of two of her pets—a dog that was mauled to death by another dog and a cat that she thought might have been killed by a neighbor. She was also dealing with multiple physical health problems, including chronic grinding of her teeth. I helped her explore the experience in her jaw muscles and show me the tension she felt in her cheeks. She acknowledged feeling angry but not wanting to externalize her anger. She identified as a peacemaker, gentle and a rescuer of animals. She said she did not want to be seen as an "angry bitch," again referring to social dictums for gender-appropriate behavior.

These two examples show how so-called "disease" can be an understandable consequence of trauma—a normal reaction to abnormal circumstances. They also demonstrate that the boundaries between health and sickness are fuzzier than a dualistic, pathology-based thinking would allow.

In contrast, the Big Health approach starts with the subjective experience and unfolds the narrative that underlies the Process. This narrative is non-linear, chaotic, unpredictable, and ambiguous. It includes Boolean logic, pathology, and the need for medical treatment. But then it goes a step further to explore the multi-dimensional and holistic nature of the person's experience and Process. From that perspective, one can be *both* sick and healthy at the same time. PTSD, IBS-C, depression, and grinding of teeth are diseases, and they are also "healthy" (i.e., normal and adaptive) responses to complicated circumstances, social arrangements, and personal histories.

Big Health steps out of a polarized medical view to present a holistic and Process-informed alternative that is not organized around opposition between health and sickness. Life is a passage through a landscape that brings us diverse experiences. Sometimes we bathe in the sun on a serene ocean beach until the wind and other atmospheric changes produce clouds, rain, and storms. We need tools to protect us from the tempests of life, and small medicine is one such instrument. Big Health accepts the small medicine toolkit but rejects the worldview of health and sickness.

Big Health and Big Medicine offer a new set of skills and attitudes that help us navigate the hero's journey across the ocean to find the Golden Fleece. Their main tool is awareness, something that travels at the speed of light and that remains constantly accessible to us. All other tools support us in developing and strengthening our awareness skills.

The hero's journey toward growth and meaning is characterized by fluid processes, developments, and evolutions. Her journey is an ongoing interactive exchange of information with her inner and outer environment. It's an endless string of experiences that will inform her own progress and that of her community. Her learning begins with a deep appreciation of her subjective experience and the feelings and thoughts she encounters along her path. Her evolution can be helped by a facilitative approach toward the phases of her process and change. I will explore these Process-informed concepts and skills in the next chapter.

In summary: Big Health and Big Medicine are non-pathological approaches to health. They do not exclude the need for pathology-based thinking to identify and treat diseases and restore small health. However, they transcend small health and pathology to explore the evolutionary and developmental properties that are an intrinsic part of any experience, especially those that challenge the integrity of our bodies, lives, and communities.

Chapter 4

PROCESS

AFEW NIGHTS ago, I dreamed I suggested to a patient that she treat her cold sore with an anti-viral cream. The next day, I felt the first tingling and burning sensations of a cold sore. I had dreamed of the symptom and experience before its physical manifestation and before I could have any awareness of it. What intelligence in me has that knowledge and awareness before its embodiment? Where does that knowing belong?

There is a mystifying Dreaming intelligence that surpass our everyday consciousness. People have used experiences such as my premonition to create theologies and beliefs in something supernatural. Science either marginalizes these realms or tries to find neurobiological explanations for them. I am taking a pragmatic approach that recognizes the forewarning dream as a Process with its own Process Mind.

Process Mind[18] is a concept that Arnold Mindell developed to describe a unifying field force and body intelligence that is the maker of our dreams. Process Mind is the incline that gives our stream of experiences its direction. It is the gravitational pull that steers our paths, lives, and processes as they follow the cascading of a waterfall or the slow meandering of a quiet creek. How do we connect to this consciousness that gives us our course, purpose, and meaning?

We are trained to focus on our momentary stationary experiences, forgetting that they are part of a larger Process or stream of experiences that continuously change no matter what. If we have faith in Process and its intelligence, then doors open. We can embrace our flaws, our illnesses, and our challenges as stages in a big-picture discovery. In this chapter, I will discuss Process Mind and other frameworks that process-oriented psychology provides. They help us understand and unwrap the individual and communal illness experience and allow us to step on the path of Big Medicine.

Conventionally, we think of waking and dreaming as two distinct states. But Process Work would suggest otherwise: like a fish swimming back and forth between the banks of a wide river (a metaphor found in the Upanishads), we meander between waking and dreaming all the time. Daydreaming, spontaneous creative thoughts, body symptoms, unintended relationship interactions, altered or extreme feelings, and impactful community and world situations are aspects of Dreaming in which we experience life through a different state of consciousness — one that is less intentional and conscious, more surreal and unpredictable.

The river's water with its currents and streams, its grounded and dreamlike experiences, is the Process. Process Work extends its methodology to include pragmatic considerations such as fixing the broken body machine while also exploring the creative significance of the experience in the moment. It overcomes the collective negativity toward illness to embrace the Dreaming of having a failing and mortal body.

There is a Taoist story of an old farmer who had worked his crops for many years. One day his horse ran away. Upon hearing the news, his neighbors came to visit. "Such bad luck," they said sympathetically. "Maybe," the farmer replied.

The next morning the horse returned, bringing with it three other wild horses. "How wonderful," the neighbors exclaimed. "Maybe," replied the old man. And the story goes on with the twists and turns of unpredictable events that at one moment appear detrimental and later turn out to be good fortune, or vice versa.

This story captures the basic principle of Process, with its motions and constant shifts in perspectives.

The Origins of Process-Oriented Psychology

Process-oriented psychology draws from Jungian analytical psychology, physics, Taoism, and many other theories. It has applications in counseling, coaching, medicine, and conflict facilitation, as well as organizational and large group work.

Carl Jung wanted to become an archeologist but chose to become a doctor because he needed to make a living. As a doctor, Jung worked for many years at the Burghölzli psychiatric hospital in Zurich. Noticing that patients' hallucinations often featured recurring characters and themes, he developed the radical idea that psychoses are not always incomprehensible but rather stories. Jung defied conventional medical thinking to see meaning in seemingly crazy behaviors and language. Looking back, he was perhaps the first Process-informed and recovery-oriented psychiatrist.

Arnold Mindell came to Zurich the day of Jung's death. He was pursuing postgraduate studies in physics at the Zurich Technical University ETH. Serendipitously, he met in a coffee shop Jung's nephew Franz Riklin, who was at that time president of the Zurich Jung Institute. Around the same time, a roommate recommended that Mindell, who was struggling with some personal issues, seek support from dream analysis with Marie Louise von Franz, one of Jung's main collaborators. Mindell was missing feelings and Dreaming in his physics studies, and he resonated with Jung's focus on dreams and synchronicity, the interplay between physical and psychological events. He began training as a Jungian analyst at the Jung Institute, pursuing the connection between physics and psychology as well as a meaning-based approach to human experience and behavior. He worked at the Institute as a teacher and training analyst while developing the discipline of process-oriented psychology, which he debuted in the early eighties.

In process-oriented psychology, every experience is part of a larger stream and is continually responding to inner and outer environmental clues. Even as some momentary experiences appear to be static and fixed, there is motion and change. Process is like a river; it has quiet and calm sections and turbulent rapids. And when you look closely, you see little churns and undercurrents in still waters and unperturbed back-waters amid whitewater. Our experiences also are fluid. Our brains and bodies are in constant communication with the environment, cease-lessly processing information and generating our lived experience. We create our own unique experience of reality moment by moment, con-structing a model of the world that makes sense. We optimize our sense of reality to function as part of a community, and in so doing disen-franchise experiences that disrupt that sense of reality.

Arnold Mindell frames this normative identity- and reality-generating impulse as *consensus reality*. This term emphasizes the fact that reality is constructed and determined by what we, as a community, agree on.

As individuals, we form our identities (and are socialized into them) through a similar process, including only part of ourselves as accept-able aspects of our identity and marginalizing what we perceive as ob-jectionable. We tend to integrate only the more culturally sanctioned aspects of reality into our sense of identity. Mindell calls this selective identity formation *primary process.*

Our primary processes include who we are, what we do, and the practical and factual aspects of our lives. The bulk of our marginalized experiences form *secondary processes* that we try to keep at bay. While they appear to us as less reasonable and rational, they are still very meaningful, enriching our sense of self, identity, and reality. Like dis-turbances in stillness, secondary processes provide deeper information.

The "crazy" narratives of psychosis, inexplicable body symptoms, fantastic dream images, and irrational behaviors of family and com-munity members come together to define an alternate *non-consensus reality*. While it is no less real and meaningful than consensus reality, we tend to marginalize it because we don't understand it enough.

Mindell took Carl Jung's interest in the extreme states of psychotic patients to the next level by integrating Jung's recovery-oriented and meaning-based approach into medicine in general, as well as into other forms of human experience like individual, group, and community conflicts.

Deep Democracy

In *The Coming Victory of Democracy*,[19] the great German novelist Thomas Mann described a lecture series he gave against fascism in 1938 about democracy as a spiritual and moral way of life. Mann saw democracy as not just a procedural or political voting system. For him, democracy encouraged the artist to seek beauty, the neighbor to seek community, the psychologist to seek perception, the scientist to seek truth. Mann's great contribution is to remind us that democracy is not just about politics; it's about the individual's daily struggle to be better and nobler and to pursue an ideal that gives meaning to life.

Arnold Mindell developed the concept of Deep Democracy in 1988. Like Mann, he expanded the classic "majority rule" notion of democracy. To deepen our understanding of life, he stressed the need to integrate both consensus reality and non-consensus-reality frameworks, voices, and experiences. To better comprehend the complete process of a person, organization, and system, we need to overcome the majority-rule principle of normative processes and include marginalized voices and experiences. Life manifests in central, primary, and consensual ways as well as marginal, secondary, and non-consensual ways. In Deep Democracy, all experiences have a voice. All are important aspects of individual and community diversity and holistic human experience.

Levels of Awareness

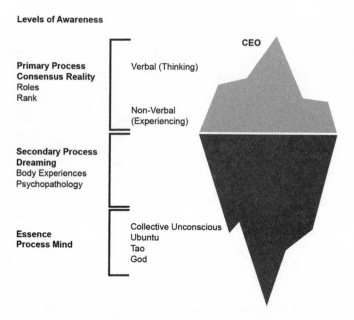

Figure 2. The Iceberg Metaphor of Awareness

Deep Democracy distinguishes between three levels of awareness (also called "levels of experience"): consensus reality/primary processes, Dreaming/secondary processes, and essence/Process Mind.

If you imagine an iceberg, consensus reality and primary processes are the part that floats above the surface of the ocean of consciousness. They are the aspects of reality that we choose to incorporate into our concepts of who we are and what we ought to do. They incorporate conventional medical views about health and normality: allopathic and even naturopathic[20] medical practices, diagnosis, and treatments.

There at the top of the iceberg, our conscious brains and minds are like corporate CEOs, focused on profit and growth. They steer the organism, emphasizing consensus reality and practical needs and avoiding unwanted emotions and unforeseen disruptions. This works relatively well until we can no longer escape their attention-seeking demands.

Below the surface are the aspects of reality that are non-consensual, that we don't want to experience. We try to push these underwater, into our subconscious, where they manifest in what Mindell calls the *Dreaming* and *essence* realms.

Dreaming experiences are the secondary processes that we disenfranchise and avoid looking at directly. They often disrupt our intentions and run counter to the goals we set out to achieve. They include puzzling night dream images, unwanted body symptoms, unexpected relationship conflicts, and disturbing altered states and community events. In teams, groups, and organizations, secondary processes manifest in conflicting roles, tensions, moods, and atmospheres.

The essence level is deeper under the water, more formless. It blends with the environing experiences of others. At the essence level, we are not sick or healthy—we are whole no matter what. Collectively, the boundaries of our individual experiences are muddled, and we become part of the common human narrative. We are both healers and sufferers, wounded and whole. At the essence level, we can connect to our Process Mind, the intelligence of many names: collective unconscious, Ubuntu, Tao, and God.

We experience all three Deep Democracy levels simultaneously, but with different degrees of awareness. For example, in this moment, my primary focus and intention is to write this paragraph. I am thinking about what I want to say, how to best communicate my message and formulate it in an intelligent and captivating way. I am sitting on my bed in the Balch Hotel in Dufur, Oregon. When I look up, I have a beautiful view of farmland and forests and, depending on the changing cloud cover, I can see the outlines of Mt. Hood in the distance. Strong winds carry rain clouds that are rapidly closing in. My primary processes are my desire to write and my enjoyment of the view outside my hotel window.

But then, my body signals me some discomfort, some strain in my lower back and some bloating in my gut. The bloating is physically not so disconcerting, but I recognize an emotional and psychological distress that accompanies it. If I pay attention to the level below conscious awareness, I can make out an inner dialogue driven by feelings of guilt about bad dietary choices and indulging in chocolate.

My secondary processes and Dreaming awareness involve both the symptom experience of bloating and the emotional reactions I have about it. Overcoming my shame, I loosen my belt and allow my belly to expand, giving space to the built-up gas. In so doing, I notice a tendency that wants my belly to contract back into a more appropriate position. I go back and forth until I understand the polar dynamics: what wants me to be more contained and what wants me to be more expansive.

As I allow my belly to take up more space, an image of a drunk with a beer belly comes to mind—a disinhibited, altered person who gives no attention to what others think of him. I am familiar with my predominant attitude of holding back, making space for others, and withholding my feelings, opinions, and reactions for the sake of keeping peace. I am less likely to blurt out my thoughts. This stands in contrast to what I imagine my inebriated alter ego would do if I gave myself the permission. My bloating brings me in contact with a whole story of restraint and conforming to familial beliefs and values that trained me in self-control.

At the essence level, I can let myself relax and let nature take its course. When I look outside the window, I see the limits and boundaries in the gullies and small ravines that demarcate the landscape and the expansions in the fields and the clouds. The scenery I see encompasses aspects of both my primary and secondary processes. There is no judgment in Nature either. As I relate to being part of Nature, I can roam freely between these different experiences and behaviors.

Deep Democracy brings attention to the multi-layered structure of our consciousness, and this increased awareness affords us greater degrees of freedom. It allows us to delve into realms below the surface of our consciousness and glean information that would otherwise remain hidden.

Escorting Clients in Their Process

Having goals of achieving better health is a reasonable attitude that we as providers and "healers" want to foster and support. In addition, we may be even more helpful if we can encourage our clients to connect with their underlying Process—the intelligence that moves them —which is unpredictable. While we need to foster hope and fight for health, limiting ourselves to this focus can obscure the information given by our clients' momentary Process. If we avoid witnessing the current experiences of our clients because they are unpleasant, we miss the opportunity to be present in the moment and help them discover something new.

In medicine as in life, certain problems are fixable; they have practical solutions. But many evade quick cures. What does it mean to support people who have issues you cannot fix? How do you provide excellent care for a client when you don't know whether they will have the stamina to face a chronic, worsening, or life-limiting problem?

Using Big Medicine and Process allows you to stay with the moment, the experience, the Dreaming—and discover the meaning. Big Medicine offers an alternative way of thinking about a client's hardships. It sees the ill and suffering person on a path of Dreaming. Treatments and cures are only partial aspects of the larger Process. Big Medicine allows you to follow the stream of unpredictable changes, to see your client as someone who needs practical solutions and also needs to connect with their Process in all of its states of impermanence. Big Medicine is about how to live a good and meaningful life no matter what comes—be it health or sickness, joy or suffering, all the way to the very end. You can help your clients do this by unpacking the flow of their Process so they can discover what makes them feel alive, present, and well. Big Medicine helps people attain awareness and true agency over their own story. Unfolding their Process helps them stay in tune with and shape their story.

Phases of Process Mind and Change

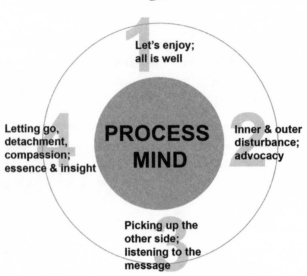

Figure 3. Phases of Process Mind

Throughout our lifespan, our consciousness develops in phases. Development, both personal and communal, is very rarely linear but rather occurs in cycles. At times we are more interested in the practical aspects of our lives, and our awareness remains absorbed with the needs of consensus reality. At other times, we are more open to Dreaming and essence levels.

In Phase 1, we stay focused on the perception that all is well and on our efforts to maintain the status quo. If we get sick or are otherwise disturbed (e.g., through a relationship conflict or community issue), we do everything in our power to fix the problem so that we can move on with our lives. We seek the help of health professionals so we can stay on track continue to enjoy what we have achieved so far. We are focused on practical consensus reality solutions and sustaining our primary process.

However, when our illness or other disturbance is more troubling and not easy to fix, we enter Phase 2, where adversity forces us to pay attention. Still, we try to keep the trouble at bay and enlist various forms of support and advocacy (from family, friends, and professionals) to maintain a sense of control over it. We pull all our fighting reserves to return to what we assume is the best for us, whether physical health or peaceful relationships. Although we feel challenged, we remain strongly identified with our own primary needs and are defended against changing our points of view. We are separate from the adversity, and we can't wait to return to the normalcy of Phase 1.

If we can't return to normalcy, or when we feel empowered enough to take our side strongly and stand for our needs (i.e., when we are able to assert ourselves as well as assume our own role in events), we may get to a place where we can start shifting our point of view and seeing the world from the perspective of the disturbance. We start to see patterns and are interested in going deeper. My recurring cold sores, for example, led me to investigate triggers such as physiological stress from wind and sun exposure as well as emotional and psychological stress from interpersonal conflicts. This is Phase 3, in which we turn our awareness to the non-consensual Dreaming level, or secondary process. Recovery and homeostasis now include learning from the illness or disturbance. In this phase, Big Health interventions help us access the information and listen to the message embedded in the difficulty. In the example of my cold sores, the information imbedded was that I needed to express my feelings and address the relationship conflicts.

The final phase, Phase 4, is one in which we can gain some detachment and perspective. We can identify with the various stages and clashing sides. We have empathy and understanding for ourselves at each phase of the journey. We value the Process for its own sake and can see the learning we have gained. In this phase, our curiosity is engaged with the organizing principles and forces behind the experiences; our common humanity and the spirit that guides us. Many spiritual traditions emphasize Phase 4 as their developmental goal: meditation and prayer prepare us to attain this phase. Process-oriented psychology values all phases as part of a natural cycle and one's Process.

The bloating Process I described above, includes aspects of all phases. In my inner work in that hotel room in Dufur, I cycled through the phases, naming the various voices and experiences associated with each specific phase: Phase 1, identifying with my focus on writing; Phase 2, noticing that I was bothered by the bloating experience; Phase 3, getting into a disinhibited, "drunken" altered state; Phase 4, connecting with the diversity I saw in the landscape outside my window. By acknowledging my inner dynamics and shaming voices, I understood the impulses that would lead me to repress the symptom and use any medical tool or medicine I could find to avoid feeling the shame. This in turn allowed me to open up to the bloating experience and discover its hidden message.

Meaning and value exists in all phases. The structural awareness in the Deep Democracy levels of consciousness and the phases of Process Mind facilitate the understanding of the Process. If you are a provider, these techniques give you an easy entry into the lived experience of a person or community, which in turn allows you to better assist them.

Let me illustrate these phases using an experience all of us can relate to: having the flu. Please, give yourself some space to explore a time when you had the flu.

Phase 1: Before you had the flu, what did your daily life look like? What were your primary goals and intentions?

Phase 2: Describe to yourself how it feels to have the flu. What were the symptoms that made you think or know that you had the flu? What do you do to try to return to your "normal" life?

Phase 3: Give the flu experience the opportunity to explain itself. Of the many experiences you may associate with the flu, choose one that is most disturbing to you, and let that experience take charge of your whole body and self. Become the flu, with its values and beliefs.

Phase 4: Imagine you can freely roam between your primary self (Phase 1) and your secondary self, discovered in Phase 3. Can you access a state of mind in which you can easily navigate between Phases 1, 2, and 3?

Big Health offers the technologies and interventions that allow us to reveal the information embedded in the disorder or disturbance. Big Medicine values the Process nature and cyclical movement of development and growth. Its ethical stance toward recovery and healing embraces the needs of all the phases. It adjusts its approach and interventions to the phase a person or group is currently in. Fighting a disease with all the armory that allopathic and alternative medicine offer is valuable — and so is using Big Health techniques and opening up to the other side.

Big Medicine helps you recognize the phase your Process is in and deepen your awareness in the moment. It supports you in your privilege to enjoy the absence of disorder and, when you do encounter some disturbance, it supports your need to complain about it and grieve the loss of equanimity. It appreciates your need to garner strength to fight and overcome the hardship and difficulty. It helps you to the other side when you are ready — and detach from it all when you need more perspective on the bigger picture.

Who, What Is the Dreammaker or Process Mind?

Now that we have examined the Deep Democracy levels of awareness and the cyclical phases of Process Mind, let us turn our attention to the underlying intelligence that informs Process. My client Jean emigrated to the country of her husband, and they have two young children. Her husband suffers from a mild form of autism spectrum disorder, and when things don't go his way, he sometimes has violent outbursts. Jean says she lives in a cage, trapped and in retreat for fear of him becoming violent during a meltdown.

For months, I approached this issue with her as one of domestic violence, believing I needed to help Jean protect herself and her children and find ways to set boundaries or leave the abusive situation. But one night, she dreamed that she was sitting in the lap of a big Buddha statue and that Buddha was intimately embracing her. She woke up feeling a huge sense of relief. Her associations with Buddha and the statue of Buddha were of feeling compassionate, solid, centered, and able to stay detached.

Jean took the dream as a guide for how to communicate with and relate to her husband. The dream also reminded her that her husband very much enjoyed sitting silently with her side by side. The dream gave Jean an answer for the relationship tension—one that was specific to her situation and more helpful than my conventional counseling guidance. Where did that Dreaming insight come from?

The Dreammaker is a symbol of the intelligence that organizes our night dreams and the dreamlike aspects of our other daily experiences, such as creative insights, body symptoms, altered states, relationship conflicts, and interactions with our environment and world. Understanding Dreaming requires us to delve into the source of our Dreaming. We can interpret dreams, unfold body symptoms, and explore their purpose and meaning; we can facilitate conflicts and community dynamics. But how do we explain the origin of and the organizing principle behind these experiences? These are existential and transpersonal issues that some people may frame as philosophical or religious questions.

In his book *The Dreammaker's Apprentice,* Arnold Mindell[21] shares how, as a child, he learned how waves are formed by the wind as well as the gravitational pull of the moon. Mindell likens the wind to our everyday consensus reality experiences that influence our Dreaming and the moon to the organizing power, Dreammaker, and Process Mind. The term *Dreammaker* refers to the uncanny intelligence that generates night dreams and creative insights and organizes our bodies. *Process Mind* is even larger, encompassing the experience of something that moves us and the universe with intent. It is a silent force, an "intentional field," a presence we can feel surrounding us and others. Mindell writes, "We find similar ideas in Bohm's quantum potential theory, Jung's concept of the collective unconscious, Sheldrake's morphogenetic fields, Reich's orgone energy, yoga's prana, and Taoism's Tao and qi."[22]

Process Mind is the source of consensus reality and Dreaming. It differentiates between the various levels of consciousness and the primary and secondary processes, and in creating diversity and polarizations brings more contrast and depth to our awareness.

If there is an intelligence in our bodies' health and illness, how can we tap into that power to use it for self-healing, learning, and growth? Doctors and healers help us to get rid of symptoms — but what if we embrace the experiences as a way to discover new territories? We all loathe to consult doctors because we fear they will tell us something is wrong, and this makes us feel bad. In contrast, Big Medicine's main value is that it sees every experience as an opportunity to get closer to the Dreammaker and Process Mind.

I believe in small health, in optimizing health and well-being — but not to the detriment of our own Process or of those who are less privileged around health. Big Medicine is more about radical acceptance of conditions, moments, and circumstances and gaining understanding and meaning. It values inner and outer diversity and the rank and privilege that come with certain experiences and the lack thereof when we are less fortunate.

If I look back at the inner work I shared above, I can see the bloating and taking space as a behavior or power that is trying to enter my life — something I could integrate as a part of an expanded identity. Another way to interpret my bloating Dreaming is to get in touch with Nature's organizing principles that create gullies as well as vast expansions. From this perspective, I can appreciate both energetic qualities — the space-taking bloating and the reactive contracting of my belly (mirrored by the openings and furrows in the fields) — as elements that come and go, that are neither good nor bad, that I can embrace or reject. The larger meaning is my connection with Process Mind, the gravitational pull of the moon.

Meaning and Coherence

For Big Medicine, healing is meaning, coherence, and connection to our Process Mind. I first encountered the concept of *coherence* through the work of the Israeli sociologist Aaron Antonovsky.[23] He had studied the resilience of a subgroup of women who had survived two major life stressors, the Holocaust and resettlement to Israel. These women had been tortured by the Nazis in Auschwitz and had lost most of their family members. They then had to build a new life from scratch in a foreign country—and they accomplished this with no major health consequences. What defined these special women was their ability to retain a sense of meaning and control in circumstances that would be overwhelming and devastating for most people. Antonovsky called this faculty *a sense of coherence*. It is a capacity to retain a perspective of life as purposeful, controllable, and manageable.

Viktor Frankl[24] had earlier stressed the importance of meaning in his own survival of the Holocaust. Even as he witnessed many prisoners lose hope and die, retaining a sense of meaning allowed him to remain hopeful and survive. For Frankl, life is primarily a quest for meaning, and a key source of meaning is courage during difficult times.

Finding a sense of meaning and coherence is what helps people overcome pain and distress. It is a capacity that promotes small health. And meaning and coherence also give people Big Health, even when their small health remains impaired. Finally, Big Medicine allows us to courageously discover meaning in difficult experiences such as sickness and disease.

Many popular coaching and counseling approaches are all about resilience and coping, i.e., "the capacity to make gold out of shit." Caring for other people and pursuing creative expressions are ways to positively deal with challenges and develop well-being. Researchers describe the health benefits of replacing a self-centered focus on the emotional impacts of our own problems with mature coping defenses and more social connections.[25] A 75-year longitudinal study of 268 male

Harvard students found that love and connection are the central factors that make life happier and more meaningful and that in turn contribute to longevity.[26] Resilience, loving relationships, and community connections are worth striving for and important factors in health and happiness.

But this attitude minimizes the importance of rank and privilege, social health disparities, and the fact that life is not always fair and controllable. Millions didn't survive the Holocaust, and most women Antonovsky studied had a weak sense of coherence and poor small health. Optimum health is a worthwhile goal—but maybe only attainable by a select few. We can learn from those who achieve it and use this learning for the benefit of others, but it will still remain exclusive. By fighting social injustice and inequality, we give people more opportunity to improve their small health and well-being. Big Medicine supports both—the fight for social justice as well as our individual attempts to increase our sense of coherence and therefore our health outcomes. It also values diversity, tensions, and health problems as openings for awareness and community building.

In closing, let me guide you through a series of small exercises that will give you an experience of the Process structures I discussed above.

Exercise: Primary/Secondary Process

1. Write down how you would describe yourself today or in this moment. "I am…"
2. Identify what bothered you today or what happened to you during the past few hours that you didn't like.

For example, I am sitting at the table and wanting to complete this chapter. I just returned from a road trip and I feel tired. Primary for me is wanting to concentrate and finish this chapter; secondary is being tired and having low energy.

Exercise: Consensus Reality/Dreaming/Essence or Process Mind

1. Describe a recent body experience or symptom.
2. Consensus reality: What practical steps did you take to deal with it?
3. Dreaming: Get into the symptom experience and discover its quality.
4. Essence: Get to the subtle pre-sensory experience of the symptom —the way it might start before becoming manifest.

Last night I had a slight acid reflux or burning experience in the back of my throat after a nice dinner. Consensus reality: I took a pill to get some relief. Dreaming: A burning sensation kept me awake. If I amplify the burning, I start to feel the excitement and passion that it contains. Essence: I imagine an almost imperceptible tickle in the back of my throat. This tickle is there to keep me awake and aware.

Exercise: Phases 1 Through 4

1. How do you currently take care of your physical, emotional, and spiritual health?
2. What phase best describes your current handling of your health concerns?
   - Phase 1: All is well, I am happy with my health, I generally don't think about it.
   - Phase 2: I have some issues that I am taking care of; my doctors or counselors are helping me manage the symptoms and keep going.
   - Phase 3: I am interested in bringing more intention to my symptoms, so I can explore them in more depth and find the intelligence behind them.

- Phase 4: I move freely between letting go, addressing the issues on a practical level, exploring the Dreaming, and staying in touch with the organizing intelligence behind all of it.

Following and facilitating Process and our attention to Process Mind, the organizing principle "heals" us and the community in a holistic way. It increases meaning, coherence, a sense of community, and Big Health. Big Medicine is about understanding the gravitational forces that pull and move us as individuals and communities. Healing (as in wellness) may be an aspect of the larger Process—but it is not the plan. Discovering Nature and Process is the larger scope of Big Medicine.

Chapter 5

INNER EMPIRICISM

~~~

To PRACTICE BIG Medicine, we need a new Process-informed language and a new way to explore the realm of our own subjective existence. Is there an empirical way of looking inward, believing in our subjectivity, and finding the answers that come from our deepest selves? In this chapter, I explore practical steps we can take to help us initiate our journey of self-discovery and healing in an existential and spiritual way.

Who are we, and where do we come from? What am I here for? What is life, and what comes after death? How do I know, feel, and experience? What is God? What was here before the Big Bang?

These are basic existential questions most of us will pose to ourselves and then shy away from. They might rise to the surface of our consciousness in the middle of the night, in times of crisis, when we are burnt out, or when we lose someone. How do we discover answers, and who determines the truthfulness of the answers we find? Philosophers, scientists, spiritual teachers, and religious scholars have debated these questions as long as human memory. Wars have been fought over them. Inner struggles keep their flames kindled. With Big Medicine, I want to show that some answers come from looking inward and what Jacob Needleman called "inner empiricism."[27]

Big Medicine is about using our inner knowledge to guide our contemplation of these questions and letting the knower in us mentor us in how we handle our own illnesses and those of our patients.

Krista Tippett, the host of *On Being*, a radio podcast about these big life questions, often asks her guests about the religious or spiritual environment they grew up in. Following her lead, I am asking myself and you, the reader, the same question because it will help us better understand our own relationship with our internal lives and truths.

Sources of Deep Understanding

Here is my answer: My French ancestors were Huguenots, or members of the Protestant Reformed Church of France (French Calvinists). Both my parents were non-practicing Christians, and we almost never went to church as a family; weddings and funerals were the exception. As a teenager, I stumbled into a more fundamentalist Christian group, wanting to remain part of a group of friends who got themselves involved with a pastor and his church. The religious practices were the background, and I continued because I enjoyed the activities and my peers.

Later I had my first "spiritual" experience in the community of Taizé, an ecumenical community in France. I was attracted to Taizé because of its deep involvement with the social and environmental lives of communities across all continents. Since the 1970s, many young adults had gathered in Taizé and shared the lives of the monks to discuss, debate, and learn from each other how to lead a socially engaged and meaningful life. This combination of social engagement and spiritual quest inspired and spoke to me.

The small village of Taizé was on a hilltop in Burgundy surrounded by large fields of rye and corn and expansive vineyards. A huge tent camp where the hundreds of young visitors lived enclosed the monastery and communal church. The house of worship was a large modernist construction in concrete with a standalone bell tower. The prayer room and space were kept purposefully bare, without pews and with candles as sole ornaments. We would sit on the floor on pillows and participate in daily morning and evening prayers that revolved around simple repetitive chants, long moments of silence, and meditative organ music. Many days, I would seek the silence of this sanctuary outside of the worship times to surround myself with the inner tranquility and peace the space provided. Sometimes an organist would practice the prayer music, and the harmonies would accentuate the feelings of serenity and soothing.

Over the years, I have yearned for the experience of inner quietness that this space and time gave me. My memories of it have changed and evolved over time. Nonetheless, they remain a source of stillness whenever I need a break from a turbulent and stressful life.

The Value of Simplicity

Simplicity is an important theme in many religions. Its value lies in helping us focus on central aspects of our lives. Through simplicity, we can gain freedom from hardship and confusion and give more attention to what is important. God is professed to be infinitely simple, and in science, the simplest theory is considered the most likely to be true. (This principle is called *Occam's razor* or *the principle of parsimony*.) Simplicity is a form of essence, and inner knowing appears to have this dimension of essence. It is often clear, unambiguous, and unifying. At its core, it is non-dual, and it helps us partake of a world filled with present-centered awareness.

Exercise: Your Source of Deep Personal Understanding

1. Identify an early "spiritual" experience that you had. What were the circumstances that helped create that experience?

2. In your mind, go back in time to that place and experience. Feel into the surroundings, the space, the sounds or lack thereof, the people who might have contributed. Let your memory recreate that experience and speak to you. Let it fill you and if you want, move you.

3. Once you feel connected with that experience express it through a gesture or brief energy sketch on a piece of paper. Give that sketch or gesture a name. Make a note of what this inner work means to you.

As I practice this inner work exercise, I visualize myself sitting on the floor of the church in Taizé. I am surrounded by the silence of that space, the light, and the chants. The sketch I draw reminds me of a ceramic bowl. I write the words "welcoming, shared silence." The practice gives me a sense of serenity, peace, and presence.

Insight and Outsight

Empiricism is rooted in the Greek word *empeiria*, which means "experience." It is a theory that grounds knowledge in sensory information. It comes from what we see, hear, smell, and taste and from what we can observe and measure. This knowledge originates in perceived events and objects from the outer world. The observations allow us to develop ideas and hypotheses in our minds that then require additional validation from our senses to become facts or truths. Science and medicine have heavily — some may say, exclusively — relied on that kind of external and objective knowledge.

Our society relegates our inner subjective experiences to the realms of psychology and spirituality. They are excluded from what is deemed real, observable, and measurable. We often think that because our subjective experiences have no direct impact on outer events, why take them seriously? Or we consider our subjective experiences to be a byproduct of our biological brains and important only as such.

We need new ideas and methodologies to fathom the science and relevance of subjective experience, the path of inner empiricism. I claim, as many others have before, that there is another way of knowing besides the one we have access to through our senses. This knowing through the senses is a kind of "outsight," focused on the outer world and the nature outside of ourselves. Having "outsight" means interacting with external reality, which has an extremely important role in our everyday lives. We must respect the validity of the path of "outsight." We need this outward orientation to function in society and take care of our everyday needs and responsibilities.

We are socialized into using our senses and empirical knowledge to conduct our lives. On the other hand, we often discount the value of having an insight-oriented language and awareness practice. We relegate inner empiricism to our religious and spiritual practices, which help us stay with ourselves and the state of Being that is bigger than us. Through the disciplines of prayer, meditation, and mindfulness, we experience our inner worlds, images, and thoughts; our breath and body feelings. These practices also teach us to detach from our thoughts and experiences, let them go, and connect more with the observer in ourselves that is not associated with the content of our observation. Our empirical outer self works as an interpreter of the content of our awareness and helps us use it.

In prayer and meditation, we get in touch with the projector that shows the movie and the screen onto which the movie is projected: We become aware of our Universal selves and the fundamental Reality and Being. Zen Buddhism speaks of no-mind, Taoism teaches about the Tao that can be said and the Tao that cannot be said, and Advaita Vedanta Hinduism centers around the idea that the true Self, Atman, is the same as the ultimate Reality, Brahman. The Christian mystic Thomas Merton said, "It is the Not-I that is most of all the I in each one of us."[28] These disciplines help us move from a perception of an outer dualistic world, in which we experience ourselves as separate individuals, to turning inward through various stages of mindfulness until we reach a non-dual realm where we become one with consciousness itself.

Empiricism in Medicine

Modern medicine has adopted a dualistic approach that separates the body from the mind, objective disease from subjective illness. By perpetuating this mind-body dichotomy, medicine looks at the body from the outside and disregards the subjective aspects of our body and its symptoms.

Looking from the outside, you measure the function of the body as a marvelous machine and find ways to repair its broken parts and pieces. Your subjective experience is deemed relevant only insofar as it gives you a warning that something might be going wrong with your machine body. It's like hearing a rattling noise in your car and suspecting that something might be broken. The car noise, or the pain that you experience after straining your back, have no significance in themselves; they are mere signals of some malfunction.

Medicine treats your body as an aspect of the outer world, as something outside of and separate from you. It disregards your subjectivity and treats your body the same way a car mechanic would handle any car. The model and the year play a role, but it doesn't matter that it is your car; it could be anybody's car or anybody's body. This mindset depersonalizes and dehumanizes the suffering human being as well as the treating physician. It also overlooks the importance of the intersubjective encounter between two human beings when one is experiencing being ill.

There are movements in medicine that seek to add a humanistic approach. Early in my career as a medical doctor in training, I appreciated the depth of understanding of the biomedical disease process and missed learning how to relate to the patient. Fortunately, I was introduced to the thoughts and practices of the physicians and psychoanalysts Michael and Enid Balint. In London in the 1950s, the couple offered a series of seminars to help physicians better understand the psychological aspects of the doctor-patient encounter and the patients' emotional experience of their illness.

Stimulated by the Balints' ideas, doctors formed peer supervision groups in which they would present "cases" and discuss the emotional content of the doctor-patient relationship. These groups emphasized learning to listen to what the patients were saying. I joined a junior Balint group of medical students practicing the art of listening and of honoring the illness stories. We focused on the relationship that was borne from the telling and listening, and we explored how to tap into the inner resources of the participants in the encounter.

Balint groups are becoming popular again, as are new approaches to medicine that include the intersubjective spaces, such as narrative medicine. These trends are part of a renaissance in medicine that is studying questions of how human beings deal with health, medical intervention, illness, and death within their social, economic, and cultural contexts. Big Medicine is part of that movement.

Big Medicine values the outer, mechanical aspects of our bodies —the ones that we want to have fixed and restored—as well as our inner experiences and subjectivity. To the outsight path, it adds an insight path of looking inward and experiencing the inner world—a world within the psyche, within the mind and the heart. It is the path of inner truth and knowing, a path that is connected to the non-dual reality. We know how to make use of outer empirical knowledge. We have less practice in applying our inner knowing for the benefit of our health and bodies. This is what Big Medicine is about.

As I am advancing in age, I notice certain changes in my body that come with what I associate with aging. My eyesight gets blurrier and my hearing diminishes slightly; at times I think my memory fails me. These symptoms, if I allow them to take over my experience, have something in common. By limiting my ability to connect to the outer world, they steer me into a more internal space and presence in the moment. They are frustrating and irritating when I try to fight them or when I feel victimized by them. On the other hand, if I allow them to be and open myself up to the experience, I am reminded of my inner life.

Many symptoms, not only the ones that come with aging, move us closer to our inner path of knowing. Depression, fatigue, and burnout are just some of many possible experiences that help us onto that insight journey. They often come to us in moments when we are one-sidedly focused on life tasks and chores and when we give beyond the savings in our emotional and psychological bank account. There is an intelligence that bestows us with subjective mind and body experiences. Can we listen to that intelligence preemptively and notice our subtle body signals that tell us to slow down, relax, and be dreamier? If you are like me, hardly ever. Mindfulness and the path of insight are good medicine in that way.

The Greek Origins of Big Medicine

Medicine wasn't always so focused on outsight. As I studied the historical context of medicine, I found multiple references that compare with the three Deep Democracy levels: consensus reality, Dreaming, and essence. I also discovered that in ancient times, medicine incorporated both an outsight and insight mentality.

The Greek god Asclepius is considered by many to be the source of Western medicine. The son of Apollo, he was raised by the centaur Chiron, who instructed him in the arts of healing. The legend says that in return for some kindness, a snake licked his ears clean and taught him secret knowledge and wisdom. That is why Asclepius is often depicted using a staff with an entwined serpent, symbolizing the power and wisdom that acts through nature. A serpent also symbolizes rejuvenation and transformation through the shedding of its skin and the dual nature of medicine that deals with life and death, sickness and health. Likewise, snake venom and other early pharmacological products were known to have both medicinal and poisonous properties.

The followers of Asclepius built temples in his honor where the sick and infirm would gather and spend the night in the holiest part of the sanctuary. After some purification rituals and other offerings, the pilgrims laid down to rest, often surrounded by non-venomous Aesculapian snakes. They expected Asclepius to visit them in their dream and give them visions, which the priests would interpret for guidance and healing.

The Greek physician Hippocrates, known as the father of scientific medicine, established medicine as a profession. He was a practitioner of the cult of Asclepius and an adept of the teachings of Pythagoras. Pythagoras is credited with many mathematical and scientific discoveries as well as influencing several philosophical and spiritual traditions. Both Hippocrates and Pythagoras incorporated nature's power and its fundamental cosmic forces into their vision of medicine.

In this cradle of medicine in ancient Greece, we find the universal principles of one force moving outward through natural and material processes and another force moving inward from dreams and other spiritual and cosmic energies. In fact, throughout history, the philosophy of medicine has at times emphasized a cosmic or spiritual God, the source of Nature, and (more recently) nature itself. Christianity emphasized that the spirit is separate from the body and nature, a doctrine that was replaced in modern science by a one-sided focus on the physical world. But at its core, medicine has that dual traction: outsight and insight.

Medieval alchemists believed in combined natural and cosmic forces that could transform base metals such as lead into gold. Nature could be tapped to develop spiritual consciousness. In contrast to contemporary science, which views nature as mechanical, blind, and void

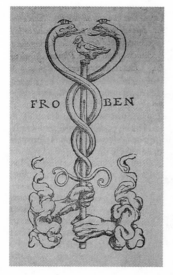

of any meaning, the practitioners of alchemy saw nature as a source for spiritual and moral growth.

Interestingly, the caduceus, which is often used as the symbol of medicine, is the traditional emblem of the Greek god Hermes. In contrast to the rod of Asclepius, Hermes' caduceus features two snakes, rather than one, winding around a staff. In early representations, the two snake heads face each other over a dove that sits atop the staff. Later, the dove is replaced by two wings. Hermes is considered the messenger between the worlds of the gods and the mortals. He carries the two essential processes that culminate in the dove, a symbol of spirit and meaning.

The aim of Big Medicine is to reconcile the naturalistic and metaphysical trends represented by the two serpents of the caduceus. It is about both using the mechanics of scientific medicine and following the dreams and visions of the spiritual realms. Through Big Medicine, we all can become alchemists and true physicians in search for meaning.

For example, every night we can enter the Aesculapian sanctuary of our sleep and let our night dreams guide our waking lives. Last night I dreamed that I was traveling to a Syrian city. In my dream, Syria was not plagued by civil war, and the city reflected the richness of its ancient cultures. When I arrived at the airport, an agent of the U.S. Citizenship and Immigration Services was issuing visas to Syrian refugees who wanted to resettle in the United States. I asked if he'd been busy that day, and he said there had been a line for a plane that was leaving for the United States. He asked to stamp my passport and I gave him my Swiss one. He noticed that my address hadn't been updated, and he scratched out the old Swiss address and replaced it with my U.S. address.

As an immigrant to the United States, I struggle with my identity. Although I left Switzerland long ago, much of my identity has remained there, in my country of origin. This dream told me to renew my home address in my Swiss passport. It wants me to keep my Swiss nature and add a U.S. address to it. I live in the Pacific Northwest, and I experience the people here as being friendlier, more open to the world, and more attuned to nature than people in Switzerland. Friendliness and connection to nature—two themes that come up frequently in my Process.

Last week I hired a Syrian civil engineer, herself a refugee, to work with the Arabic-speaking refugees I help resettle. Yesterday was her first day at work. My night dream wants me to visit the historical, political, cultural, and religious richness of that part of the world. What does this mean? Although I work with other individuals from that part of the world, I haven't yet taken the time to truly visit with them and appreciate their deep cultural contributions.

How do I relate the meaning of my dream to my body and its health? When I think of Syria and its civil war, the civil war in myself over my sense of personal identity—of feeling at home, my heart—comes to my mind. I sometimes worry about the health of my heart. I have no heart condition, but at times I feel slight cramps in my chest. I also worry about my cholesterol levels and fear I could die of a heart attack.

My Swiss nature makes me a diligent and effective worker, and I fear that the stress caused by working so much could ultimately weaken my heart. Unconsciously, I put a lot of pressure on myself and treat myself harshly. I understand Syria as being a rich melting pot of cultures and religious beliefs. I work with and serve many individuals and families from that region, and I also embody a cultural ambiguity within myself. My heart is the container that holds all these thoughts and feelings. If I follow last night's dream, it directs me to bring more friendliness into my world and to enjoy nature. Unfolding my fear of a heart attack, I let myself succumb to death and return to Nature. In that state, I experience a sense of stillness and pure being.

Hermes the messenger, with his winged sandals, moves freely

between the worlds of the gods and the mortals and is the guide to the underworld. He is the mediator between the conscious and unconscious, the inner and outer; he guides our inner journeys. His healing powers are symbolized by the staff he carries, the caduceus. The two serpents stress our need to maintain a constant connection with our visible and invisible worlds, to employ both outer and inner empiricism.

In medicine, employing outer empiricism means consulting health professionals, taking care of our emotional and physical needs, exercising, eating a healthy diet, and complying with recommended treatments. Outwardly taking care of my heart, I exercise, minimize my intake of bad fat, take a baby aspirin daily, and reduce stress.

Hermes tells us not to stop here, but to continue our journey and turn our attention inward, into the realm of the underworld, the subconscious, the spiritual. This requires us to use skills of self-observation and inner attention. It forces us to stay with our feelings, thoughts, body sensations, dreams, and altered states. As we follow Hermes into the underworld, we begin to learn how to embrace Hades, the god of the underworld—a form of our inner divinity. To really live, we need to embrace death. Our mini-deaths, the illnesses that remind us of our vulnerability and looming mortality, are part of Hermes' healing force. My own heart's inner journey links me to nature, friendliness, and an internally focused state.

Quantum physics tells us that matter has two simultaneous forms: a particle and a wave. Explaining the nature of light, Einstein wrote, "We have two contradictory pictures of reality; separately neither of them fully explains the phenomena of light, but together they do."[29] Medicine has strong expertise in the world of particles and has led us to neglect the wave world, which involves a different form of being and knowing. For us to relate to our wave nature, we need to open ourselves to nonmaterial parts of ourselves—our dreams, altered states, intuitions, fantasies, and our irrational thoughts. Waves are unbound by matter, transgressing the boundaries of our bodies. They connect us with each other.

In the illustration of Hermes and his caduceus, the heads of the two serpents face each other and enclose the dove. The snakes can be seen to represent two principles we've discussed: consensus reality and Dreaming. The dove then stands for a third principle, the essence level or spirit.

To illustrate the essence level, I think of leavening. In the past few months, I have been fascinated with baking sourdough bread. I have always been a bread baker. During a gap year from my medical studies, I spent six months on a remote farm in the Jura mountains of Switzerland. My hosts were Mennonite farmers who followed strict values of ecological and sustainable agriculture. They had a wood oven in which once a week we would bake bread for the whole family. With them, I learned the basics of bread baking.

Later I would bake Zopf for Sunday brunches, a braided white flour bread with an egg yolk glaze. Until now I never dared to bake sourdough bread, knowing the challenges of creating a starter, making the leaven, and proofing the bread for the right amount of time. Reading Michael Pollan's book *Cooked*[30] inspired me to give it a try. Our ancestors in Egypt discovered about six thousand years ago how to process grains from grasses using the natural fermentation process from the leaven that had captured the naturally occurring yeast and bacteria. The leaven turned the rudimentary porridge into something that was bubbling with air and life and that, when cooked, became a wholesome bread. This more nourishing food contributed to Egypt's transformation from a hunter/ gatherer culture to an agricultural society.

Baking a loaf of sourdough bread is an alchemical process and experience. Sourdough is alive, and as the fermenting organisms transform the wheat into a more digestible and nutritious food, they help the wheat realize its potential. For me it's a metaphor for the transformation that can occur when we concentrate on our inner life and let it inform and direct us. Our inner lives are the leaven we need to grow and expand. It helps me better understand why Jesus, in the gospels of Matthews and Luke, compares leaven to the realm of God and heaven.

Our inner alchemical process brings inner fermentation and transformation.

Blaise Pascal writes in his *Pensées* (139): "I have discovered that all the unhappiness of men arises from one single fact, that they cannot stay quietly in their own chamber..."[31] We ask the questions I listed at the beginning of this chapter. Yet their answers remain elusive to our intellectual understanding. They are questions of the heart and soul and therefore require a different interpretation.

Intuitively, we know that there is another world beyond the one we perceive through our senses. Past the outer appearances and beyond the realm of particles, there is an inner world of experiences and direct sensations in which we are more wavelike; a world that transgresses the boundaries of the material realm. As Pascal found, if we remain focused on the world outside, if we avoid our inner chambers, we risk depression and burnout.

The sourdough leaven needs to be cultured and nurtured. Half of a batch of leaven is used for the loaf of bread you intend to bake, while the other half is kept aside and fed with more flour and water to be replenished. Our inner worlds require the same process of nurturing, feeding, and replenishing. The practices of inner work, meditation, prayer, and mindfulness are how we nurture our leaven. Here is a very easy exercise for feeding our leaven.

Exercise: Replenishing Your Inner Leaven

1. As you sit, relax your shoulders and your neck area and let your mind let go of its focus.

2. Notice your breathing and take a few minutes to track your inner experiences. Observe inner images, sounds, body sensations, and subtle movements.

3. Stay with these experiences and let them guide you. Notice the images, sounds, body sensations, and movements; track their natural progress as they change. Follow your stream of thoughts and experiences and see where they take you.

4. Make notes about what you have discovered.

As I engage in this short inner work exercise, I notice my body's tendency to want to collapse. Following that impulse, I begin to see myself as a wooden puppet with strings attached to my limbs. Above me is an invisible puppeteer. My forehead is illuminated by stage lights. I meditate on this image.

My attention is drawn to the powerful mystery of who is directing the movement of my wooden limbs and what is shining light onto my existence. My inner Dreaming images reflect an inner existential quest about what moves me and the source of my creativity, awareness, and purpose.

Inner empiricism gets us in touch with our Process. It enables us to step out of the automatism of everyday life and connect with aspects of ourselves that remain hidden from our everyday consciousness. What we experience gives us access to an alternate and deeper reality. In my normal state and identity, I am not in touch with parts of myself that are collapsed, lifeless, and without energy. In turn, if I allow space for the collapsing Process, my attention shifts to the puppeteer and the light, and it brings me to the threshold of what may be a spiritual journey.

Chapter 6

BIG MEDICINE FOR
PATIENTS AND PROVIDERS

⤳

THERE IS A tradition in the Swiss Alps that, if you leave your front door unlocked, you allow anybody to come into your home, where they will expect to be served coffee. My friend and mentor Arny Mindell has spent a lot of time in the Swiss Alps. His extraordinary interest in people and his relationship skills have given him insight into Swiss mountain culture and practices. One of his friends, Fritz, a hermit and alpine farmer, had special abilities to commune with nature. He would hunt foxes by waiting until he sensed their presence and then chasing them into traps. Fritz would also show up unannounced, and if the door was unlocked, he would step into Arny's kitchen and expect to be served coffee and schnapps.

Big Medicine teaches us to believe in our own subjective experiences, to have faith in our own Processes, and to invite unknown guests to step into our home so that we can build relationships with them. Big Medicine is also about communing with Nature, getting closer to the Dreammaker, connecting with our Process Mind, and unlocking our inner essence.

If you are a patient who is struggling to cope with an illness, Big Medicine gives you practical steps for learning to relate to the guest that has stepped into your home. If you are a provider, Big Medicine helps you develop a sense of curiosity toward the numinous aspects of your patients' struggle with illness.

Starting from the awareness of your inner essence, it follows your Process—the doors that are open and the doors that are locked. It welcomes both familiar and estranged experiences and invites them to the coffee table to be valued as part of our journey toward awareness. It also respects the need to lock the door sometimes and keep the unwelcome stranger, such as illness and suffering, away.

As Antonovsky[32] states, we are all chronically ill, continuously struggling to cope with the onslaught of challenges to our bodies and health. In bell curve medicine, the goal is to skid back under the bell curve and restore an ideal state of health or normalcy. The problem is, health challenges constantly recur, we are forced out from under the bell curve, and then we blame ourselves for failing to stay healthy. Big Medicine recognizes that health and sickness are part of an ongoing Process, a never-ending dance between different states and experiences. Rather than an idealized state, individual health is from a Big Medicine perspective our ability to fluidly move with the Process and *commune* with the powers and forces of Nature as they engage and test us.

Communing

Communing is a deep and intimate way of relating to a person, a spiritual entity, or Nature. I am using this verb to illustrate a specific way we can relate to our own body or, as a health professional, to a patient's body process. Philosopher Eugene Gendlin spoke of *felt sense*, which he explained as "a special kind of internal bodily awareness ... a body-sense of meaning"[33] that the conscious mind is initially unable to articulate. The neuroscientist Francisco Varela coined the terms *embodied action* and *embodied cognition* and concluded that "organism and environment enfold into each other and unfold from one another in the fundamental circularity that is life itself."[34]

As we engage in transformational interactions with the world, we participate in it: We enact the world and are shaped by it. Communing is a specific way of getting in touch with our embodied experience and its relationship to our environment and context. To deeply understand our embodied actions and cognitions, we need to explore the levels of experience that I have introduced: consensus reality, Dreaming, and essence.

Communing begins with understanding the existential threat that any unwelcome body experience provokes. Unexpectedly, we become aware of a disturbing body feeling and sensation. This creeping or some-times sudden experience pulls at our awareness and we begin to scrutinize its meaning and potential danger. We compare it to previous sensations and draft a plan of action to address it so that we can return as quickly as possible to the comfort of our usual unburdened state of being. The stranger is not welcome, and our main strategy is to get her out the door as quickly as possible.

Depending on the problem, we might enlist the services of allopathic and alternative health professionals, over-the-counter medications, bodywork, acupuncture, chiropractic, herbs and supplements, prescription drugs, and maybe even surgery. We approach the issue from a practical point of view, identifying its causes, meanings, and the best ways of getting rid of it so that we can go on with our lives.

At this stage of our engagement with the guest, we are, as in Arnold Mindell's Phase 2 of process and change, fighting the disturbance. To open up to the experience would be, in this developmental phase, too dangerous and too disruptive to our everyday lives. It would require us to face and confront our vulnerability and ultimately our own mortality. Often, this fighting approach is successful, the illness is cured, and we are able to return to Phase 1 and move ahead as if nothing had happened. Phase 1 and 2 are also the arena of bell curve medicine. We use all the tools of bell curve medicine to get rid of the uninvited visitor or body symptom and prevent her from returning.

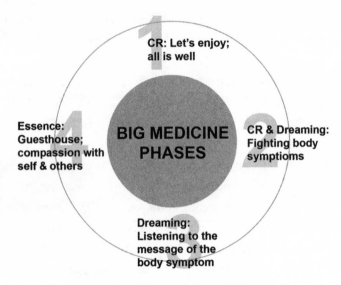

Figure 4. Phases of Big Medicine

Deep down, we know this is not going to last—we will eventually have to meet the stranger and face our mortality. We also all know people who don't have the same privileges of good bell curve health and who are dealing with chronic illness and early death. But it is easier to live with a cognitive bias of invulnerability and illusory superiority. Psychologist David Myers termed this the *Lake Wobegon effect*, defined as the human tendency to overestimate one's achievements and capabilities in relation to others. This phenomenon is named for the fictional town of Lake Wobegon from the radio series *A Prairie Home Companion*, where, according to host Garrison Keillor, "all the women are strong, all the men are good-looking, and all the children are above average."

Big Medicine invites us to move beyond Phase 1 and 2 and our refusal of the uninvited visitor. For this, we must have the courage to engage with our body experiences in a way that includes both the fighting and an interest in getting to know them more deeply. Opening the door to an unwelcome experience is extremely difficult, and nobody can do this all the time. It is okay to wander the roads of Lake Wobegon. But with some support and encouragement, we can find the audacity to move to Phase 3 and let the visitor in so that we can get to know her and learn from her. This starts with turning our attention to the subjective experience of the body symptom with at least some amount of openness toward exploring it candidly.

The language and symbolism of our body symptoms is associative and dreamlike. This is the reason why Phase 3 is also called the "Dreaming level." Unfolding Phase 3 starts with turning our attention to the subjective experience, scrutinizing the specific qualities and making them more easily accessible. This we do through amplifying the subtle experiences by, for example, breathing into the area of the body where we experience the symptom. Another way is to imagine a symptom maker, an agent that is creating the symptom in us, and then get into the head and mindset of this symptom maker.

You may recall how I helped Martha, the car accident survivor from Chapter 1, to enact both the car that caused the accident and the pain maker that caused her shoulder injury. Unfolding the Dreaming qualities of the body symptom and exploring its subjective meanings gives us an alternative point of view. Not unlike opening up to an opponent's point of view in a conflict, the act of debating with the uninvited body symptom incites us to discover a new perspective and worldview. For Martha, this worldview was one of a newly empowered professional woman.

Communing with body experiences goes beyond welcoming and becoming acquainted with an uninvited guest or estranged part of ourselves. In Phase 4, at the essence level, we unite with our primary or Phase 1 identity, which wants to live life unencumbered, and we also unite with our secondary or Phase 3 identity, which has a different purpose and meaning. In Phase 3, we stop acting like Procrustes and cease to align ourselves with mainstream expectations; instead, we open up to our own diversity. In Phase 4, we not only welcome visitors, we also become Procrustes' guesthouse—but a version of such that welcomes everybody and doesn't cut down their limbs to fit the bed. This is a phase in which we embody a general attitude of welcome and unity with whatever and whoever crosses our path.

In his poem "The Guest House," Rumi exemplifies the Phase 4 essence attitude: "This being human is a guest house. / Every morning a new arrival. // A joy, a depression, a meanness, / some momentary awareness comes / as an unexpected visitor. // Welcome and entertain them all! ... Be grateful for whoever comes, / because each has been sent / as a guide from beyond."[35]

The essence or guesthouse attitude is one of eldership. The elder has lived a fulfilled life and lived through most experiences. She knows it all, as in she has a lived experience of the ups and downs and twists and turns on the road of life. Paradoxically, the most difficult mental states —grief, burnout, depression, thoughts of suicide, and fears of impending death—can be powerful means of connecting us with Phase 4, our essence level. These experiences, unabated, pull us down and inward into the body of mother Earth. They awaken us to existential questions about our purpose and reasons for being alive. They are potent doorways into becoming both the elder and the guesthouse.

To experience the various phases of communing with a body symptom, try the following exercise. You can do it on your own or with a helper.

Exercise: Communing with a Body Symptom

Choose a body symptom you have experienced or are experiencing now that, in your mind, has the potential to cause death. Or choose an imagined symptom that could kill you.

Phase 1 or Consensus Reality:

1. Describe your primary identity, which is your normal state of being. In other words, what is your personality like in general, and how do you usually go about everyday life?
2. Make a brief energy sketch on a piece of paper of this primary state of being. An energy sketch is like a doodle or scribble that captures the quality of the experience.
3. Look at that sketch and give it a name.

Phase 2 or Fighting:

1. Name the body symptom that in your mind could be fatal.
2. Remember how it felt or feels, or imagine how it would feel.
3. Describe how you fight it and how you try to make sure it doesn't return.

Phase 3 or Dreaming:

1. Concentrate on the symptom experience, the region of the body it upsets until you have a good sense of how it feels.
2. Imagine a symptom maker, the entity that is generating the symptom in you and that could recreate this experience in someone else.
3. Make an energy sketch of the felt quality of the symptom or of the mindset of the symptom maker.
4. Look at the sketch and give it a name.
5. Go back and forth between being your usual self of Phase 1 and embodying your secondary identity, the symptom maker, of Phase 3.

6. How does it feel to embody your Phase 1 identity? How does it feel to embody your Phase 3 identity? What are the differences between them?

Phase 4 or Essence:

1. Imagine the symptom actually killing you. How would it achieve this? Is it a slow destruction of your body self, as in cancer, or a quick choking of your vital energy, as in a stroke or heart attack?
2. Why would the symptom maker want to kill you? Does she have a message she wants to convey that you could use in life?
3. Now let yourself be killed by the symptom quickly, and imagine and explore death. Suddenly, you are dead. Where does your soul go? What happens to you?
4. Follow that experience until something in you relaxes.
5. Explore that experience and make a third energy sketch that encapsulates that state of being. Give it a name.
6. From that state, look at how you could integrate the symptom experience into your usual life. Let your imagined death give you some advice for how to go about your life.

I used to have asthma, and I am still identified as an asthmatic. I always carry an emergency inhaler in case I suffer an asthma attack, even though it has been years since I had symptoms. Asthma is scary and, as most know, potentially deadly if untreated. So, let me use this as an example to illustrate this exercise.

Phase 1, Consensus Reality: I am usually pretty mellow and go about my life at a rhythmical, routine, and tempered pace. My moods are in the middle range with some bouts of mild depression and fatigue. The energy sketch I am drawing is like a slow to moderately paced tune composed of eight notes in the middle range of the scale with some lower notes. The name I give is the sketch is: rhythmic flowing tune.

Phase 2, Fighting in Consensus Reality: Over the years I have had two severe asthma attacks and many milder asthma-like symptoms. I experienced the attacks as wheezing, pressure, and choking in the middle of my upper chest, like a strong hold and gagging of my upper airways. For years I have used an emergency inhaler and a daily cortisone-based anti-inflammatory inhaler.

Phase 3, Unfolding the Dreaming: My asthma feels like a fist is pressuring my sternum or breastbone and squeezing my upper airways tightly in its grasp. It's controlling the air that is flowing in and out of my lungs. My focus and attention are fully drawn to that experience, and I lose track of my surroundings. It is as if I am pulled inside of myself. I am powerless and in the hands of my asthma.

The sketch I draw is circular with strong strokes around the middle and a downward motion. I name it "inward focused power and strength." In musical terms, it is a series of unmodulated whole notes in the lower register. My imaginary impersonated asthma maker is a warrior who is holding me down by the sternum and telling me to stop moving so I can get in touch with my core self.

As I meditate on these primary and secondary experiences, I recognize that in my functioning at work, I am pulled by my tasks, duties, and chores to the point where I lose contact with myself and what moves me. I am mostly outwardly oriented—I'm motivated to help my clients, manage the programs I oversee, and problem-solve all the questions my co-workers bring to my attention. I very rarely take time to daydream and be with myself.

However, in my asthma state, I am forced inside; I have no way to escape from the hold that pressures me to feel my chest, my lungs, and the air that struggles to go in and out. The doer and helper in me wants to do a good job and support my clients and teams. The asthma side of me is more interested in the deep feelings and insights that arise from the silent depths of contemplation. When I play music, I am more in touch with this part of me, which I otherwise tend to marginalize. The question now is, How can I live my life more intensely from the inside out, supporting the doer while also staying in tune with my inner self?

Phase 4, Uncovering the Essence: I do suspect that my asthma warrior could potentially kill me in her chokehold. Her intent and message are unmistakably clear: She wants me to be true to my inner life. If I let her choke the air out of me, I stop breathing and become still. I close my eyes and my whole body lets go. My attention is drawn to an inner light that I perceive in the upper-right corner of my right eye. I let myself be pulled toward the light, and I merge into it.

The sketch I draw is of a bright star with a dark core. I name it "sunflower." The sunflower is both radiant and still. Its yellow petals are alive, moving in all directions, while its center is dark. My sunflower moves its head with the sun to stay connected with this source of energy.

I imagine living my life as a sunflower, both movable and still, in contact with the enlightening sun. As a sunflower, I am present but less active at work. I share my insights and knowledge but I am less tempted to be proactive and reactive and solve other people's problems.

Big Medicine for Providers

If you are a healthcare provider, Big Medicine will enable you to connect to your patients' experiences in a holistic way. Your patients will feel deeply seen, heard, and understood, and it will help you build sustainable relationships with them. But let me start with an email I read on a listserv I am linked to:

> I've been in the hospital for a few days for a relatively simple surgical intervention for my gallbladder. Here in the hospital, it is a desert for the heart. Feelings are not welcome here, and I suffer additional emotional pain and solitude because of that. It's so frustrating and painful trying to have a decent human relationship with doctors or nurses. They are inaccessible, no space to really listen, no help if you ask and you want to understand what's going on in your own body and what they are doing with it. It's as if your body

94

and your health is not your business, you shouldn't ask, only wait as silently as possible. I think it's just brutal, these attitudes, and I notice it not only with me but as a general attitude with patients and their families.

There is such a rank disparity with no awareness at all around it. They abuse their rank, and there is a complete marginalization of feelings happening all the time. This is really painful, and it doesn't help the healing process. No surprise that people's faces here look almost always so serious, unhappy, and sad. Today I have particularly suffered for that.

There is so much work to do in the world and for sure the healthcare system needs a huge, important updating.

The grievance this email is expressing is one that is widespread. Healthcare professionals are often unaware of their rank and power, dismissing the feelings and subjective experiences of their patients. But then, I would argue that we all contribute to the failings of our healthcare system. Together we are stuck in consensus reality and Phases 1 and 2 of Process Mind. This bias forces healthcare professionals to narrow their focus to fighting disease using objective scientific tests and tools. Most providers, especially physicians, are not trained in how to attend to the whole person; nor are they willing or even expected to do so. They have a specific task to fulfill, and it doesn't encompass subjective feelings.

In contrast, Big Medicine opens to the realm of subjectivity, connection, and spirit. As health professionals, it gives us powerful relationship tools and helps us move beyond the mere fighting of disease in Phase 2 and relate to the whole person.

To relate to the whole person, we must with understanding and recognizing the power dynamics between provider and patient. But this topic deserves a broader space, so I have dedicated an entire chapter to it (see Chapter 9).

Here, I want to focus on what Big Medicine can offer us in our roles as professionals and providers. First, disease is not Public Enemy Number

One anymore or at the top of the Most Wanted list. Sickness and health are a Process we participate in. Our role changes from being the soldier against disease to being a co-facilitator of a multi-phased process with multiple protagonists: the patient (or client) and her family, friends, pets, and co-workers, as well as her dreams, visions, values, and social and cultural identities.

The Process evolves on a stage. As providers, we can help direct, choreograph, and participate as actors improvising within the Process. The Process gives us broad stage directions that we can try to follow so we can unravel and express their meaning. Providers play an important role as protagonists in the drama, helping our co-actors bring out the essence of their characters.

Who we are as artist providers is essential to our craft. We have unique styles and feeling skills that are a key part of our facilitation. I can best explain what a feeling skill is by describing the way I play saxophone. I can learn the technical skills of having the right embouchure, playing the scales, knowing the chords, and following the rhythm. Besides these technical skills, I will play in a certain timbre that is unique to me. This sound is linked to the specific anatomy of my mouth, throat, and chest, as well as to my personal musical sensibility. In human interactions, we have both "technical" skills (i.e., good communication skills) and feeling skills. The latter are like presence. We can use our feeling skills as interventional tools with our patients, offering them our presence as supporters, facilitators, and witnesses. When we combine our technical skills with our feeling skills, we can play our one-of-a-kind music.

Amy Mindell[36] coined the term *metaskill* for the feeling skill that each individual brings to her practice, be it art, counseling, teaching, or medicine. Many clients and patients seek our services not only for our knowledge and expertise but also for the healing that our metaskills can offer. As we interact with the whole person across from us, her experience of her story is influenced by our facilitator style and charisma. Our metaskills can help or harm the client, acting as placebos or nocebos.

Metaskills have powerful effects. In my book *Health in Sickness,*

Sickness in Health, I dedicated a whole chapter to the placebo and nocebo consequences of our attitudes and implicit messaging. Placebo effects are the therapeutic benefits that result from, for example, harmless sugar pills and from the positive suggestions and expectations that a clinician gives his patient. Nocebo effects are the opposite—the harmful outcomes that can stem from clinicians' negative beliefs.

As we communicate either hope or gloom, we hypnotically induce physiological changes in our clients' and patients' bodies. The metaskills we employ in our relationships with our clients and patients are powerful tools that can foster healing and cause damage, so we must use them with care.

In summary, our materialistic and factual approach to disease is beneficial from a Phase 2 perspective; we can help our patients fight. But with its implicit reduction to the diseased and broken machine body, we constrain our clients and patients to believe that they, too, are also broken and diseased. None of this is true or the whole story. From a Big Medicine perspective, your patient is neither sick nor healthy, broken nor whole. She is on a lifelong Process journey.

Exercise: Metaskills

1. As a provider or caregiver, think back to some moments when you've received positive feedback, praise, or compliments about your personal style from a client, patient, friend or family member you were helping. Choose one of those compliments that you feel describes your personality or unique style. Write it down.
2. Amplify this metaskill to get to its core value by feeling into it.
3. How much do you recognize yourself in this newly discovered core value? How much do you marginalize it in your work with clients/patients?
4. Set an intention to use this metaskill very consciously with your next client/patient.

Many of my clients appreciate the calm, non-judgmental space I provide, in which they feel safe and welcome. This metaskill reminds me of my favorite beach on the Oregon coast: Strawberry Hill. The beach is protected by a small cove lined with spruce trees and ferns. Lava rocks and large tree trunks populate parts of the beach. In one section of the beach, I often find agate and other gemstones.

In my work, I often feel pressured to achieve certain outcomes. To justify medical necessity, I am obliged to develop treatment goals and document their progress. If I imagine embodying my Oregon beach nature, I relax and can hold both myself and my client with our agendas and needs. Like the beach, I have no judgment and can appreciate the overall Process with all its implications and requirements. I can focus on discovering gemstones.

Learning about your metaskills and becoming more conscious about community issues are the building blocks of fostering trusting and sustainable relationships. (For a larger discussion of the community issues I am referring to, see Chapter 8.) They help improve client and patient retention and compliance with your recommendations. Using a Big Medicine approach will help you stay in tune with your visions and aspirations and prevent burnout.

As providers, we are told to abstain from personal disclosure and focus on the needs of our clients and patients. We learn that the moral and ethical thing to do is to keep clear professional boundaries and avoid building personal relationships with our clients and patients. We are in a more powerful position, so crossing these professional boundaries can lead to an abuse of power that hurts the persons we are here to serve.

Although I agree with this recommendation in general, I do believe that for health professionals, one important form of self-disclosure can help establish good relationships with our clients and patients: our transparency about our own health issues. A few weeks ago, I attended a public dinner. A woman sitting across from me suddenly started choking and spitting food and saliva. Panicked, she ran out of the room. As I had experienced similar events in the past myself, I recognized what was happening. She was still breathing normally, so nothing was stuck in her upper airways. I knew she was experiencing a spasm of her esophagus.

I followed her out, explaining to her that I was a doctor and understood what she was going through because I'd had the same thing happen to me. I told her I had gone to the ER several times and that on my last visit, a nurse had given me a great trick that helped immediately. I gave the woman a sip of Coke to hold in her mouth as long as she could without swallowing. In the warmth of the mouth, the carbonated gas expands and slowly stretches out the esophagus. Once she was no longer able to keep the Coke in her mouth she should forcefully swallow it. This technique worked and relieved the woman from the painful and scary spasm.

My self-disclosure helped me establish a trusting relationship with someone I hardly knew and facilitated a situation that required both calming and speedy intervention. Disclosing your own experiences with being sick and in pain can be very beneficial. It shows that you have some understanding of what your client or patient is going through. The danger is that you could make your own experience the standard. This is not the idea. Use your personal examples with caution, and don't make your client feel bad if their experience is different than yours.

In professional relationships, we are not supposed to reveal ourselves. People seek us out primarily for our professional skills or our institutional role and not for us as people. By crossing the boundary of self-disclosure, we redefine the relationship and open the door to expectations of more friendship and intimacy. Add in the power imbalance inherent in the provider-client relationship, and disclosure becomes potentially unsafe. We are not our clients' friends and confidants. When it comes to the issues they consulted us for, we are not their equals.

However, the experience of illness is isolating. Patients are thrown out from under the bell curve, their identity changes, and they may feel victimized. Despite the support of family and friends, their journey with illness can be a mostly solitary road of uncertainty and suffering. As practitioners, we can strengthen the therapeutic bond with our patients by disclosing our personal experiences with illness, our vulnerabilities and limitations. Yet because of the inherent power imbalance and the risk of influence, we must approach personal disclosure carefully. When contemplating a personal revelation, we need to consider our intentions and weigh the risks and the benefits. Disclosing our own issues may diminish the importance of our clients' own processes.

Self-disclosure is unavoidable. We can't hide our gender, age, skin color, foreign accents, health status, and physical abilities. We reveal ourselves through many visible and invisible signals, such as tone of voice, body language, moods, how we dress, the setup of our office, and how we greet our clients. Our feeling skills, or metaskills, expose our personalities. Everything we do speaks loudly about who we are; every intervention is a signature that reveals something about us.

We as professionals can be both facilitators of healing and barriers to healing. There is still little knowledge about what makes a good therapist or health professional. Technical skills and professional knowledge are obviously relevant, but they are not the whole story. Relational skills, empathy, collaboration, the ability to build alliances and adjust to feedback, diversity consciousness, and rank awareness are some of the soft skills that have an impact on outcomes.

From a Big Medicine perspective, as providers, we are entering another's story with our own story. The client, with his story and needs, is requesting support. Sometimes that support is just about needing our technical skills for help in combating the disease. He is in Phase 2 and fighting hard, and he wants nothing more than to return to his normal life. At other times, especially if the illness is prolonged or more threatening, he might need more intentional emotional support. The isolation of being sick and the existential threat to his ordinary identity creates a new dynamic. Suggesting a change in perspective and attitude, offering a Process view, and abstaining from using a pathological approach can help our client develop a new relationship to what until now was merely victimizing him. Can we join our client in Phase 3 and help him make sense of what is happening to him?

Recall the example of Martha, the car accident survivor from Chapter 1. I was able to work with her a third time, and this time she chose to explore her insomnia. Since her two accidents, she has struggled with falling and staying asleep. She used to be a good sleeper, and the chronic insomnia was adding an additional burden to her recovery and sense of wellness. More recently, she'd had surgery on her shoulder, and the brace she was required to wear made it impossible for her to sleep in her bed, so she had to sleep in a reclining chair. Just talking about it, she became very emotional and communicated her deep suffering and pain.

I asked her why she wanted to sleep. Besides the obvious reasons, she mentioned also yearning for quietness and traveling to another world in which she could dream. Next, I asked her what stood in the way of her getting to that state. She switched into another voice to tell me that sleep was overrated, there was no time to sleep, she wanted to play more, and there were many important political and cultural issues that needed her attention. She shared that, since her accidents, she was just getting her energy back and feeling able to accomplish certain tasks. She now felt pressured to be more productive, and this stress was hindering her sleep.

We role-played her two conflicting needs and clarified some of the details of her ambivalence. I then asked her to step back and watch me playing out both sides of this conflict, while her task was to find some resolution. From a more detached vantage point, she identified the struggle between doing and being. She recalled how her brain injury had forced her to stop working so hard and learn to be more in tune with her momentary energy levels. She remembered the medicine that had helped her be with herself—a particular practice of art making. Since her strength started coming back, she had abandoned that valuable practice. I suggested she use that same medicine before going to sleep.

Approaching sickness with a Big Medicine narrative, as patients and providers, we are co-creating a meaningful story. Our dialogues uncover an experience, a story, a meaningful Process that evolves in phases.

There are times when we just want to live our lives and not be bothered (Phase 1). Then something starts to trouble us (Phase 2), and when we can't avoid it anymore, we have to address it. We seek help and hope to get rid of the unsettling experience. Often this works, and we can go back to pursuing our undisturbed lives. Occasionally, symptoms persist and we are compelled to explore the deeper meaning (Phase 3). Big Medicine helps us navigate all the phases and uncover the Dreaming experience and essence (Phase 4). As in an artistic process, Big Medicine facilitates how we apply color, contrast, and value to the canvas so we can bring out the underlying images that wants to be exposed. Each phase reveals different shapes and forms, none superior to the other.

Chapter 7

THE INNER EMPIRICISM
OF COMMUNITIES

⁓

NOW THAT WE have explored Big Medicine for individuals, I want to shift the focus to communal and public Big Medicine, first by looking at the inner worlds of communities. Like individuals, communities are formed by visible outer worlds and social forces as well as invisible inner worlds and field forces (which I will explain below).

Social, political, and cultural structures inform the development of our communities. They determine power hierarchies, moral codes, what we are taught in school, how we sustain our material existence, how we restore health, and more. Systems of social rank and power dynamics ensure that some people have better access to financial resources and health than others. To counter these inequalities, civil rights, women's rights, and other social justice movements fight to help us achieve more egalitarian and just societies. Academic disciplines like social psychology and economics study social dynamics and behaviors. All of this remains largely in the realm of empirically accessible outer knowledge.

The inner life of communities surfaces through their histories, stories, visions, and values; in their tensions and conflicts, in the extreme states of its most marginalized members, and in the ways communities respond to environmental processes. (Many psychiatric patients deemed "delusional" share their fears, albeit in extreme ways, about how new communication devices are invading their privacy. California just experienced terrible wildfires. Local community members and firefighters responded heroically, showing the best side of humanity. In contrast, a certain politician faulted regional forestry practices while denying the effects of climate change). The inner worlds of communities are also shaped by field forces that influence perception, behavior, and communication. Gestalt psychologist Kurt Lewin studied the interaction between a person's psychological state and his or her social environment and vice versa.

Lewin described how individuals internalize external stimuli from the physical and social worlds into their own "life space." Like fields in physics, external signals from the community create an unconscious field force that influences the behavior of community members. Intrinsic aspects of individuals, interpersonal dynamics, and inherent systemic forces determine the field, which in turns affects whoever enters the field. This field, this hidden force, is something beyond the outer empirical world. Like a magnetic field, it polarizes and creates diversity of behaviors, opinions, values, communication styles, and roles.

To ground this discussion in an example, in most social groups I am quiet, listening more than I speak. However, I am also part of a certain professional group in which I frequently find myself making jokes. The tension and competitiveness of the group brings out another side of me that I typically would not identify with. In another group that I'm part of, one member has strong views that she repeatedly expresses to the point of annoying other members. But if she misses a meeting, someone else will represent her point of view. These are examples of this organizing field: the interpersonal dynamics create an almost magnetic pull that influences how I behave. The phenomenon of social fields is being examined in studies of group dynamics, conflict resolution, and organizational development.

Diversity is an integral aspect of life. It manifests itself externally in cultural and social identities as well as internally in the conflicting viewpoints and identities we can hold even within ourselves. One person may even hold diverse and conflicting social roles, such as physician, wife, and mother.

Without external and internal diversity, there is no consciousness and awareness. Differences create polarities that help us, when we process them, to become more aware and to grow. Systems of oppression continuously leverage elements of social diversity—such as race, class, gender, and sexual orientation—to disempower, marginalize, and minoritize some people while elevating others. Thus, diversity is used to create hierarchies and grant or limit the access of individuals and communities to resources and opportunities, including health outcomes. ProPublica and NPR reported recently about one appalling example of health disparity: Black women in the United States are three to four times more likely to die from pregnancy-related causes than white women.[37] Such unjust dynamics create trauma and suffering and must be stood against.

However, in our secondary, Dreaming experiences—night dreams, body symptoms, altered states, and the roles we embody in groups and conflicts—we all share most aspects of diversity. In these secondary experiences, we take on identities outside of our usual selves. The figures in our night dreams, for example, personify all sorts of characters and behave in all sorts of ways. This gives us a base to develop some understanding of the others' lived experience and build community.

Rumi wrote: "Out beyond ideas of wrongdoing and rightdoing there is a field. I'll meet you there. When the soul lies down in that grass, the world is too full to talk about." Throughout our lives, we do each other right and wrong—we hurt each other, and we heal and reconcile. Then, Rumi invites us to reach out to the field itself and rest on its grass. The field is now a power that is more than one created by humans and their environments; it is one with its own intelligence and one that has many names: Allah, God, essence, Process Mind, and the Dreammaker.

The outer world is full of injustices and disparities that we need to fight against. But then, this outer world, and the communities that make up this world, have inner experiences. These inner experiences include the emotions revealed in conflicts, protests, festivals, and celebrations, as well as in art, music, and architecture. Each of these experiences has an inner drive, purpose, and Dreaming that aspires toward a collective transformation. We express these stories in values that drive our community alliances, such as political parties, churches, and other groups we affiliate ourselves with. By joining these groups, we often keep ourselves separate or tribal and disenfranchise the "other."

But Rumi's field is the underlying ground on which we can meet each other. With our souls, we can commune with the field, momentarily step out of the world, and reconnect with our common humanity. Michelle Alexander, a civil rights lawyer and author of the book *The New Jim Crow*, said in an interview with Krista Tippett that stillness is an act of our public selves, allowing us to connect with a revolutionary love:

> And I think for me what it means to be fully human is to open ourselves to fully loving one another in an unsentimental way. I'm not talking about the romantic love, or the idealized version of love, but that the simple act of caring for one another, and being aware of our connectedness as human beings, and the reality of our suffering, and the reality that we make a lot of mistakes, and we struggle, and we fail.
>
> That's all part of being human. We suffer, we love, we struggle, we fail, and then we love again. And I think trying not to imagine that we're anything more or less than that, as human beings struggling to love and find our way, making mistakes, but still yearning for a deeper connection and a sense of purpose in our lives is what being human is all about.[38]

The stillness of meditation and prayer helps us connect with what it means to be human and resist the fear-driven impulse to divide and marginalize. In this space, on this field, we can see the world honestly and soberly. We can wake up to our current social, political, racial, and environmental realities and acknowledge our own contributions to them. As Alexander explores in *The New Jim Crow*, we are all "sinners" and criminals; we break God's laws and human laws, and we transgress moral and ethical values, in varying degrees. Acknowledging our complicity—that most of us break the law not once but repeatedly throughout our lives, and that we all fail to live up to our ethics and values— makes us humbler and more human. It also entails the recognition of our own limitations, the small nature and divisiveness that keeps us closed to the other, and our inborn preference to belong to a small tribe of people that look like us, think like us, and share the same values.

Alexander also observes that the most punitive nations in the world are also the most diverse. We are more punitive towards those we view as "other"; the United States incarcerates brown people at staggeringly disproportional rates. Diversity is challenging and brings out polarizing forces. But let's face it, we all find it challenging to accept our own inner diversity, and inside, we hold on to a sense of identity that is tribal in nature. No wonder that our communities have the same challenge. With age and maturity, we start to recognize the multiple facets of our identities and become elders, individuals who have lived through a lot and have experienced themselves in a range of diverse roles and identities. The elder is a role we need both internally in ourselves and outwardly in our communities. We can find our inner elders by cultivating our internal spaces as individuals and communities.

Assigned social ranks and memberships based on skin color, gender, sexual orientation, age, class, size, and health are like a river that flows in one direction, consistently advantaging the same people and consistently marginalizing the same people. Social ranks give some people unearned privileges and withhold those privileges from others. They are based on false and arbitrary categories. They dehumanize everybody, both marginalized people and those with more rank and privileges.

Promoting slogans like "we're all one" without acknowledging the reality of social disparities can prolong oppression. If we are a member of a privileged group, our desire to be inclusive may lead us to think we understand a marginalized person's experience. But this presumption hinders our ability to simply be with the pain and suffering of another person's oppression. Thinking we know what is going on for someone else disrupts our ability to witness what is going on for him or her. Wanting to extend the sense of oneness may be motivated by a hidden agenda of wanting to stay in our comfort zone.

On the other hand, most of us are members of a social group that experiences some degree of marginalization, be it because of our age, gender, race, sexual orientation, religious affiliation, immigration status, class, physical ability, size, primary language, or other difference. This gives us some partial knowledge and experience of discrimination. Even so, we can't assume this gives us expertise about someone else's experience, and it is better to place the sense of understanding in that person rather than in our own interpretation of his or her experience. As health professionals, teachers, helpers, and facilitators, we are in the business of making change possible and are often pressured to achieve some outcome. We must be aware of the danger of discounting social ranks, being exclusive and perpetuating marginalization. When we work with individuals from a marginalized group, we need to stay humble and open letting them guide us (except for instances where they endorse attitudes of internalized oppression).

For example, I currently coach an aging gay man who feels isolated and depressed. He engages in the diversion of brief paid sexual encounters he finds through Grindr, a gay dating app. He can't afford them, and they don't make him feel good about himself. As a straight man, I must be careful not to go along with his own diagnosis of sexual addiction, which carries a taste of internalized homophobia. Helping him with his "sex addiction" could cause harm in enabling homophobia. I need to learn more about the complex social norms of sex in the gay community, as well as about the cultural oppression that older gay men experience.

Big Medicine incorporates inner empiricism on both the individual and community level. The subjective, internal worlds of individuals and communities are as real and impactful as the external worlds. Inner and outer experiences overlap and intersect, influencing each other. Knowledge of and expertise in inner experiences is required to deeply understand individuals and communities. Growth, long-term change, and liberation hinge on our ability to navigate our internal and external worlds.

Big Medicine asks us to learn the new language of inner experiences. Anyone who has learned a new language knows the intricacies of absorbing new words, concepts, grammars, and structures. The language of inner knowing helps us communicate more intimately with ourselves and with others. Effective change and understanding comes slowly, in phases, and with humility. Big Medicine wants us to be permissive and nonjudgmental with ourselves and each other so that we can build true community, which comes only with knowledge of the history and painful effects of discrimination across social groups. At the end, we can become allies for each other and develop a felt sense that we are each other.

Chapter 8

BIG MEDICINE AND OUR SOCIAL AND CULTURAL ENVIRONMENT

⤳

THE KITARAS ARE a family of Afghan refugees. They recently resettled in the United States after living for five years in a refugee camp in Pakistan. Three older single daughters stayed behind in Peshawar. They haven't been granted refugee status and are being persecuted. They keep calling the parents in the middle of the night, begging for help. The three younger siblings and their parents, who are safe, are tormented by the fear for their sisters' and daughters' safety.

Not long after arriving in the United States, the father had a disabling heart attack and stroke. The mother suffers from kidney problems, and the three younger siblings are missing school to take care of their sick parents. The medical case managers for the Kitara family are getting increasingly frustrated because they feel the parents are not taking enough care of themselves and are neglecting their children. What to do?

In this chapter, I explore how our social and cultural environment —the way we treat each other and structure our communities—influences our health. Social marginalization, the unequal distribution of resources, and racial and gender discrimination create physical symptoms and suffering. Big Medicine explores not only the role of individual health issues as valuable experiences for inner awareness and outer change, but also the importance of social justice issues as challenges and solutions for community health.

How does Big Medicine inform our day-to-day practice, both as patients and providers? Big Medicine for the community attends to all levels of society: the individual, the community, and institutional and social systems. It addresses individual experiences and contributions and develops their meaning in both a personal and community context. It continues with the individual in relationships and explores various interactional dynamics. Further, Big Medicine techniques can inform the facilitation of small and large groups using education, training, group forums, and community discussions. Big Medicine also confronts structures and systems of oppression that contribute to health disparities and other social ills.

Unequal social and cultural arrangements affect people living in these environments through all the phases of Process Mind: consensus reality, Dreaming, and essence. As I discussed in Chapter 4, Deep Democracy explores the multi-layered and cyclical aspects of individual and community experiences. It encompasses reality-based approaches, feeling-based interactional dynamics, and moral, ethical, and spiritual perspectives. Big Medicine uses the methods and values of Deep Democracy to promote awareness and process community change and growth.

The Kitara family exemplifies the web of individual and community issues that affect people's health. Their story is one of war, trauma, and political and ethnic conflict. They have dealt with labyrinthine international refugee and immigration policies, the systemic oppression that causes health disparities, and the challenges of maintaining individual coping skills and resilience.

Health Disparities

In the documentary *The Divide*, public health expert Michael Marmot relates a stark example of a social context that is shortening people's lives.

> In Glasgow, men living in the poorest parts have a life expectancy of 54. In India, three-quarters of the population live on two dollars a day or less. No one in Glasgow lives on two dollars a day or less, and yet men living in the poorest parts of Glasgow have a life expectancy that is eight years shorter than the average in India. And I thought: 'Aha, that's it, that's going to explain it:' being relatively disadvantaged has profound consequences, which determine high rates of suicide, violent death, alcohol, heart disease.[39]

"Relatively disadvantaged" is Marmot's key point: Poverty is not the only factor causing health disparities. It is also important how you fare in comparison to people around you. If your neighbor is much wealthier than you, you are likely to be less healthy than your neighbor—and you also may be less healthy than people who live in far more deprived circumstances than you but who have neighbors living just like them.

Returning to the road trip metaphor from Chapter 3, we are not mere life tourists attempting to drive away from the dangers of disease and injury. Rather, we are participants in the co-creation of our journey toward health. As co-creators, we also have a collective impact on the health journeys of others. Our social contracts, including the distribution of wealth, affect the health of marginalized and privileged individuals and communities. These systems sculpt the terrain that marginalized people travel. As a society, we don't just give some of us less robust means of transportation for navigating life. We bar some entirely from access to health mechanics; we sabotage their cars and throw nails in their paths.

Big Medicine for individuals explores how human beings deal with health, medical intervention, illness, and death. Big Medicine for groups and organizations examines the social, economic, and cultural contexts of health, illness, and healthcare. It does this while adhering to the three levels of consciousness that form the Deep Democracy framework. On the level of consensus reality, Big Medicine takes a public health approach and addresses the social structures that affect health and its equal or unequal distribution. For example, Martin Daly and Margo Wilson, two evolutionary psychologists, studied income inequality in Chicago's 77 neighborhoods. They used the Gini coefficient, a statistical measure of wealth distribution, as a measure of wealth and income inequality. They associated this coefficient with male life expectancy at age 15 and male-to-male competition, dominance, and homicide. They found a life expectancy difference of 24 years between the richest and poorest neighborhoods. Inequality and relative poverty was also associated with life expectancy in women and a tendency for women to have more children and have them earlier. Relative inequality increases the levels of stress hormones such as cortisol, which leads to more aggression and disease. The amount of certainty and uncertainty in people's environment shapes their thoughts, choices, behaviors, health, and life expectancy.[40]

At the Dreaming level, it unravels the community relationship dynamics and the stories that shape the community's identity. At the essence level, it considers the moral, ethical, normative, and spiritual dimensions that provide communities with meaning and direction.

In the case of the Kitaras, our team intervened first to help them with their immediate practical needs. Before they could really address their trauma, they needed to get home care so their younger children could go to school. We then engaged the community by linking the Kitaras to the local nonprofit organization Portland Meet Portland, which links refugee families with mainstream volunteers. Their case is not an isolated individual story, but one that speaks of the suffering of so many refugees around the world—and one that deserves to be shared and carried by a whole community.

Individual Versus Collective Wealth

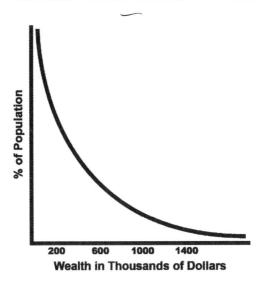

Figure 5. Pareto Curve Showing Distribution of Wealth

Previously, we discussed the normal or bell-shaped distribution of health. Wealth and income have a different distribution, called a *Pareto curve* after the Italian economist Vilfredo Pareto. The Pareto curve shows that the highest percentage of the population has low levels of wealth, while the lowest percentage of the population has the highest levels of wealth. This is a reason why governments use gradual tax rate increases to partially redistribute income. Other social programs, such as Social Security, Medicare, Medicaid, food stamps, and subsidized education are in place to compensate somewhat for what many perceive as a rigged game.

This wealth distribution graph is an example of a collective pattern. Some people contend that income and wealth success is based on individual merits, such as responsibility, work ethic, and intelligence. This individualistic view holds that we are each unique and that our social group memberships (i.e., those based on race, class, and gender) are irrelevant to our opportunities. It claims that there are no intrinsic systemic barriers to individual success and that the failure to realize

115

the American dream is the fault of individual character, not of social structures. But we know that group membership is important—that, for example, being socialized as a man is a different experience from being socialized as a woman, and that to be a woman in a male-dominated culture comes with negative consequences.

One can also argue that in many instances, treating an individual for a health condition is a failure of prevention. Research into public health has demonstrated that the social conditions in which people are born, grow, live, work, and age influence how they think, how they respond to stress, and how they cope with trauma—and that this, in turn, profoundly affects their risk of physical and emotional illness. Many studies have proven a direct link between adverse childhood events, abuse, and traumatic stress and long-term negative health outcomes and early death. Microaggressions from everyday prejudicial interactions and macroaggressions from sustained systemic racism, sexism, and other forms of social marginalization have similar negative effects.

Under chronic stress, our brains produce higher levels of stress hormones, which in turn affect multiple physiological processes, such as our immune response, or sugar and fat metabolism. Our bodies' sympathetic nervous system, which controls our fight-or-flight response, keeps us in a state of hyperarousal if it is chronically turned on. The logical consequence is a gradual wearing down of the body's healing abilities and the eventual breakdown of our bodies.

Adverse conditions such as poverty, insecure jobs, and lack of agency in their work impact people's sense of empowerment, as well as their access to resources and money, which in turns worsens their health. These social disadvantages are among those that make and keep people sick at a higher rate than those who are more privileged and in control, resulting in stark health disparities. Put simply, the unequal distribution of privilege creates an unequal distribution of health outcomes. For example, studies of health in residents of various Baltimore neighborhoods showed a 20-year difference in life expectancy between those living in the most disadvantaged area, Hollins Market, and those living in Roland Park, the most wealthy and privileged part of the city. The mere fact of being born in one place can give you an average handicap of dying 20 years sooner than your more privileged neighbor. Only six miles separate the two Baltimore neighborhoods, but this can determine if you live an average of 20 years longer or not.[41]

In fact, the cumulative impact of our inequitable social contracts actually kills people—a factor that is rarely included in common mortality statistics. We read about changes in death rates from heart failure, cancer, suicide, and motor vehicle accidents. We don't read enough about the early death that can result from living in impoverished neighborhoods.

The Politics of Health

Society and health are highly political. Some claim that in a meritocratic society, everyone can overcome social difficulties and that it is not the role of the state to provide welfare for poorer individuals. Others point to individual lifestyle choices as contributing and relevant health factors.

These arguments may sound logical, but they ignore the fact that people cannot take responsibility for their actions if they have no control over their lives. The data shows that social determinants are causes of unhealthy lifestyle choices. Whether or not people receive sound health advice does not correlate with how they will behave in the future and what choices they will make. Very few people eat healthier or exercise more because their doctors tell them to do so, when their life circumstances are not conducive to such choices.

Both absolute and relative poverty cause poor health. Poverty forces people to live in environments that make them sick and limits their access to healthcare. Being poorer than your neighbor adds an additional burden of comparison that creates emotional stress and ill health. These are the reasons why people living in poverty are more likely to die of substance use, diabetes, hypertension, and obesity.

In my view, it's irresponsible to speak of personal responsibility when social structures result in health disparities that kill people. Putting the blame on the individual prolongs the criminal negligence of failure to address health inequities, and it allows the more privileged to remain comfortable and unquestioned. As Karl Marx wrote, "Men make their own history, but they do not make it as they please; they do not make it under self-selected circumstances, but under circumstances existing already, given and transmitted from the past."[42]

Health inequalities are, as Michael Marmot showed in his renowned Whitehall study,[43] about everybody, not only the poor. Researching the health outcomes of British civil servants, Marmot demonstrated that the social health gradient involves everyone, from the bottom to the top of the social ladder. The higher your position on the ladder, the better your chances to stay healthy and live a long and productive life without disability. As discussed above, the issue is not just absolute poverty but also relative poverty compared to others in your surrounding environment. This is why men in Glasgow live on average 8 years shorter than their counterparts in India even though they are much richer.

The levels of poverty and the magnitude of inequalities across the spectrum of social structures are what create health disparities. Increased opportunities for education and jobs, along with the sense that our voice and participation are valued by our society, are factors linked to good health. Generally speaking, the access you have to money and other resources relative to others is a prime influence on your feelings of empowerment, security, control, and dignity; your freedom to be and to do; and your chance to stay healthy and live a long life.

Relative poverty, relative dignity, and relative respect all speak to a relational comparative process among individuals in a particular community. Health disparities hinge on how we share privileges across the social gradients and how we deal with aspects of our communities' diversity. Addressing absolute poverty means redressing inequalities and injustices. Addressing relative poverty means increasing the voice and participation of disenfranchised individuals to improve the health of the entire community.

Freedom of Choice

The economist and philosopher Amartya Sen examined social choice and social justice issues, such as the freedom we have to lead a life that we have reason to value.[44] He assessed social arrangements by their effects on actual lives. He found that people's capabilities depend not only on their physical and mental characteristics, but also on their social opportunities and challenges. Thus, he concluded that the real measure of well-being is not just people's actual functioning or their level of satisfaction with their lives, but also their capabilities—the set of options from which they can choose.

For example, the high school graduate who is waiting tables has an unmistakable advantage over the high school dropout who is waiting tables. Both function, for the time being, at the same level. However, the high school graduate has more choices. The same is true for the mountaineer who suffers from frostbite; he is obviously more advantaged than the homeless person who freezes out of necessity.

Sen saw freedom of choice as an essential ingredient of well-being. He also understood that well-being is a kind of freedom—the freedom to lead a life that we value. That privilege depends both on real opportunities and on a sense of freedom from constraints and challenges. This means that people's health and well-being depend not only on actual circumstances but also on the amount of freedom they perceive they have to make choices.[45]

As we all know, behavioral differences contribute to health inequalities. Unhealthy eating habits, smoking, and lack of exercise are health factors that differ across individuals in a population. But patterns of behavior are also conditioned by our living and working environment. One study found that individual behaviors accounted only for about one third of the participants' adverse health outcomes, whereas environmental/social factors were the main reasons for poor health.[46] Especially for people at the bottom of our social status ladder, the process of comparing themselves to others activates the body's stress, inflammation, and immune responses.[47] Social insults act like physical threats. Our bodies' crisis management systems are designed to respond to the immediate danger, so they prioritize immediate short-term gains over long-term interests. The threats of inequality and marginalization are long-lasting and lead to chronic stimulation of our bodies' stress responses at the expense of our future health and life expectancy.

As the gap between the rich and the poor increases in the United States, poor white people are experiencing what people of color have experienced for a long time: the emotional and physical stress of ongoing microaggressions from feeling worse off in comparison to others. Our ability to feel well, physically and emotionally, depends on how we choose to live—and those choices are strongly influenced and determined by our social contexts and environments. We can see poverty as an environmental pollutant that limits early childhood intellectual and social development, therefore also limiting physical and emotional well-being. As a society, we should work to remove the "toxin" of poverty wherever possible, just as we have removed lead and asbestos from our homes.

Trauma's Impact on Health Disparities

The Kaiser Permanente Adverse Childhood Experiences Study (mentioned in Chapter 3) found a direct correlation between the number of traumatic events a child or community experienced and the emotional and physical fallout these events caused: the greater the trauma, the longer the ensuing emotional and physical distress would last.

The combination of poverty and adverse childhood and community experiences makes children, individuals, and communities more vulnerable to illness. Chronic poverty and traumatic events activate the body's biologically embedded stress response, which involves the hypothalamic-pituitary-adrenal axis and the autonomic nervous system. This stress response is mediated by the body's emotional regulation centers (e.g., the amygdala and the locus cerulean), and it impacts the development of memory, social affiliation, and other executive functions.[48] Furthermore, recent studies in the emerging field of epigenetics demonstrate that social environment and interactions are able to modify human DNA and the subsequent manufacture of proteins.[49] Social inequalities and traumas have a direct physiological impact on the body that can be engraved in the DNA and transmitted over generations.

Let me share an extreme example of the direct health consequences of adverse childhood or community events. Twenty-one years ago, Lask and colleagues first described a condition they called *pervasive refusal syndrome* (PRS).[50] They described it as a child's "dramatic social withdrawal and determined refusal to walk, talk, eat, drink, or care for themselves in any way for several months" in the absence of an organic explanation. In recent years, refugee children in Sweden have been responding to the denial of their families' asylum applications with *resignation syndrome*,[51] a condition in which refugee children give up on life. They slowly retreat into an unresponsive and apathetic state that can last for months. They fully depend on external care, artificial nutrition, and other medical support.

Researchers have tried to explain PRS in a variety of ways since Lask first described it. They have categorized it as a form of post-traumatic stress disorder, learned helplessness, "lethal mothering," loss of the internal parent, resignation syndrome, depressive devitalization, and a primitive freeze response. In the case of the refugee children, some have suggested "manipulative" illness, meaning the possibility that the children have been drugged to increase the family's chances of gaining asylum. Others have insisted that PRS is simply depression, conversion disorder, catatonia, or even a factitious condition. Basically, the cause is poorly understood. But it demonstrates the powerful implications of extreme stress and hyperarousal of the bodies' crisis management systems.

The refugees, with their histories of severe emotional and physical trauma and their experiences of post-traumatic stress, rightfully conceptualize their experience as a natural reaction to unnatural circumstances.

Most funding of health benefits is focused on the individual and relies on individual symptoms and conditions. But trauma, as discussed earlier, is not only an individual but also a collective experience. Our diagnostic manuals don't include a community-based post-traumatic community stress disorder.

Part of trauma-informed care is to provide advocacy and culturally sensitive services. Refugees and immigrants in the United States can lose their rights for obtaining legal status if they are found to be a "public charge" who is utilizing government support or who is likely to seek government services in the future. At the time of writing, a draft proposal of the Trump administration seeks to expand this public charge policy to include the access of federal health insurance benefits, Social Security, and other federally funded programs for the poor. The immediate consequence of this draft proposal is that many refugees and immigrants are not seeking services and support, for fear of jeopardizing their immigration proceedings. This is putting their health in danger. To mediate this injustice, my colleagues and I are participating in advocacy efforts to combat this policy change.

Low Rank and Trauma

Being of low rank,[52] or of low relative social status compared to others in our immediate or larger environment, is another type of trauma or chronic microaggression that results in the breakdown of our bodies' crisis management systems and can lead to ill health and early death. These are normal reactions to unnatural causes and social arrangements. When we treat an individual who suffers from obesity, hypertension, and diabetes with the understanding that these conditions are co-created by the individual's social environment, we confront the limitations of our current individual-based medical thinking and systems. Diagnosing and treating individuals for the consequences of collective trauma and adverse social arrangements is insufficient. We need a new community-centered medical framework: one that treats the individual, addresses the root social causes, and tries to repair the social damage.

Differentiating between states of health and disease allows us to identify physical wrongs so we can develop treatment solutions. Similarly, social polarities, tensions, and inequalities bring forth social ills, and they also increase our awareness of the consequences of systemic oppression. They help us understand the impact of social and relationship dynamics and how rank and power differences not only marginalize people but also make them ill and eventually kill them. To say it bluntly: Inequality is probably a bigger killer than any disease.

In the United States, the Civil Rights Acts and the Americans with Disabilities Act prohibit discrimination in serving marginalized communities. Providing language access is one way of being non-discriminatory. But until now, nobody thought of requiring pharmacists to label prescription containers in consumers' primary language. For the refugees we serve, this led to frequent misuse of medication and deleterious health effects. To address this issue, my colleagues and I have worked with nursing students who participate in their public health rotations with us to draft a legislative concept that addresses this obvious systemic problem. At the time of writing, this proposed new law will be introduced in the next session of the Oregon State Legislature.

Democratic decision-making processes trust in the intelligence of the majority of a group or community—but they marginalize the voices of those who are in the minority. However, a greater awareness about diversity and inequality is facilitating the development of social medicine, a community-based form of medicine that integrates a public health and social justice lens. Social medicine has the potential to spur debates, the development of new community relationships, and changes in policy.

Deep Democracy and Eudaimonia

Big Medicine and Deep Democracy respect democratic institutions and processes and aim to foster a deeper understanding of people's emotional responses to social structures, systems, and interactions. From a community perspective, Phase 1 describes a stage in which a community is socially indifferent, taking refuge in the sanctuary of its own privileges and distancing itself from the pain felt within other communities. Polarization and diversity characterize Phase 2 of a community's development. Although troubled by conflict, Phase 2 allows us to deepen our understanding of individual and collective trauma, and it serves as a starting point for change.

Change comes not only through democratically chosen transformations but also when individuals and communities begin to put themselves in the others' shoes and walk in them. This typically requires a facilitated community dialogue where individuals and groups can speak out, stand up for their diverse points of view, and be supported to hear others out and find spaces where they can relate to the opposing views. This is Phase 3 of a community's development.

Deep Democracy includes an ethical and moral stance, one that aligns with the Greek philosophical term *eudaimonia*, which translates to "human flourishing." From a modern philosophical perspective, eudaimonia can be understood as a felt sense derived from poise, wisdom, and an ethical way of life. High levels of eudaimonia are synonymous with an increased feeling of purpose, along with greater levels of social integration, personal growth, social contribution, and autonomy. In modern psychology, eudaimonia links to individual and community self-actualization and well-being. A community ethics, wherein individuals and groups can both stand for their position and remember that we all have a shared human experience (Phase 4), helps us overcome differences and polarizations. It goes beyond a democratic approach, which marginalizes minority views.

Intelligence Beyond the Intellect

To follow an ethical way of life, we must rely on several different human faculties. We need *emotional intelligence*,[53] [54] which combines the capacity for empathy with the ability to work through emotions and conflicts. We also need *communal intelligence*, the ability to understand the values and dynamics in community relationships. Communal intelligence requires diversity consciousness: participation in the community, knowledge of the diversity and other social factors that organize the community, and the willingness to step outside of our own comfort zone and relate to opposing points of view. Communal intelligence also entails a respect for differences and a recognition of the unequal privileges and powers associated with disparate social positions.

The term *communal intelligence* contains the word *commune*, which emphasizes a deeply felt exchange among individuals and their environment.[55] A person with communal intelligence takes a moral and ethical approach to community relationships and is able to see the community lucidly, with its harmonious aspects as well as its polarizations and inequities. They believe in the inherent wisdom of communities and aim to facilitate their community's awareness and its future growth and wellness.

To tap into communal intelligence, we must find detachment and take a wider perspective. For some, this comes from an ethical or religious place; others find it in nature. We can also utilize our own embodied awareness by relaxing our mind, letting our body be moved by its own knowing, and exploring our Process Mind.

This ethical aspect of communal intelligence can only be temporary. It is a phase in an individual's[56] growth and journey. Communal intelligence includes the understanding that in a natural cycle, a moral stance will be replaced by a phase of renewed conflict and polarization.

The notion that community growth is cyclical, moving through the four phases of Process Mind, allows for a non-pathological understanding of community dynamics. Like individual ill health, social disparities and inequities are, as well as being grave injustices, opportunities for awareness and evolution. When processed and facilitated, they can foster growth and a deeper understanding of diversity.

In May 2017, two young Muslim women were harassed by a white man in a Portland train car. Three men stepped in and were stabbed by the perpetrator. Two of them died. The agency I work for was asked to emotionally assist the two traumatized young women and a friend of the perpetrator. Big Medicine starts with helping the individuals on all sides, but it doesn't stop there. In response to this tragic event, we also supported other groups of Muslim women in processing their heightened fear and anxiety, we launched a series of educational and training events for community health providers, and we are developing several community dialogues and open forums. Big Medicine advocates for health justice and social justice and fights to overcome avoidable health inequities. The health gap and other disparities between the rich and the poor threaten the stability of our communities. Big Medicine doesn't stop at this public health perspective. It continues with exploring the individual and relational implications of social justice issues. To get a personal experience of this, try the following exercise.

Exercise: Social Justice Awareness

1. What is the social justice issue that upsets you most at the moment?
2. Identify the various players involved in this issue and imagine the viewpoint of each one.
3. Which viewpoint is most disturbing to you?
4. Explore that perspective and its various talking points. Then feel into its energetic quality.
5. Express that energy in a gesture or hand motion. Make a quick sketch of that energy.
6. Where would you locate that energy in your body? Do you have any symptoms in that area?

7. Explore your viewpoint on the issue. What do you stand for? How is your viewpoint affected by the opposing perspective?

8. Express the quality of your viewpoint in a gesture and energy sketch.

9. Now, tap into your deeper wisdom. Find a mindful big-picture perspective. You can do this, for example, by going in your mind to a place in nature that makes you feel whole. Look at both sides of the issue. Can you discern within yourself a communal intelligence that can identify with both sides?

10. Imagine drawing on that communal intelligence as you interact with someone who holds that disturbing viewpoint.

11. What changed?

12. Now imagine using your insights in a community education or dialogue project.

I am upset about the increasing gap between rich and poor in the United States and the unequal access to so many resources. What infuriates me most is people who state that they deserve all their privileges. I am distressed by their self-image of having earned their financial and professional successes as a result of their own efforts while ignoring the complex social dynamics that contribute to their privileged positions in society. I feel this side is entitled and arrogant.

To explore that perspective, I walk around, feeling into it. I notice myself walking more firmly and with purpose. The gesture that goes with it is one of strength and tightness, my hand making a fist and asserting itself. Relating this energy to my own body, I am reminded of various symptoms that I sometimes experience: asthma, a tightness in my chest, an esophageal spasm that happens to me when I eat dry food too fast, and my anxiety about having a heart attack, which I also imagine would come with a painfully tight cramp.

As a health and social services provider, I aim to help those who are ill and socially underprivileged. This side stands for equality, universal health, and justice. The gesture that captures this point of view is one of embracing and cradling.

To access my ethical intelligence, I let my mind relax, and I move following my body's own impulses. The motion is one of slight drunkenness with wavelike movements and random quick spurts. It reminds me of the ocean, which has smoother waves out farther and crashing waves where the water hits the rocks along the shore. Engaging with the entitled role, I connect with the ocean sprays and feel a sense of elevation and pride. Relating to my own pride, I can support my antagonist to express, believe in, and appreciate his own pride and sense of achievement.

If you are a provider, Big Medicine is here to help you develop trusting relationships with your clients and patients. Trust builds on emotional and communal intelligence. And trust builds on relationships. At my workplace, our communally intelligent clinicians come from the communities we serve. They share a common refugee story and attend the same churches and mosques. They often volunteer in community health clinics or other community-led organizations. For people who come from a more dominant culture, creating these relationships is even more important.

Again, emotional intelligence is your ability to understand your own feelings and empathize with another's feelings and experiences. Communal intelligence is your ability to, in Process Work terms, desegregate yourself from the exclusivity of your historical and social space. Each of us has our own story, our own historical and social context. We all grow up in a more or less segregated social milieu, meaning that we are socialized to think in certain ways and behave according to values and norms that are based on attributes of race, class, gender, religion, and sexual orientation. We then tend to think our experiences are universal and become blind to the differences in culture and subculture. As healthcare providers, we develop unconscious biases and may fail to understand the challenges that our clients and patients face in complying with our interventions and recommendations.

For providers, a first step toward developing communal intelligence is to unmask the disparities by "disaggregating" your own experiences from those of your patients. In research, to disaggregate data is to break it down into smaller units, which allows the results of the studies to be analyzed for their effects on demographic subgroups. It helps to capture the distinct experiences of diverse cultural groups.

To personally disaggregate your own information means to reclaim your culture, unique history, and lineage at the same time as you model diversity consciousness. For example, I am privileged in terms of race, class, gender, and sexual orientation, but I am marginalized in terms of age and primary language. Disaggregating is about becoming transparent about the social positions and privileges or lack of privileges that come with each specific identity.

We are all more or less rank unconscious when it comes to our identities and their unearned privileges, but we are likely all too aware of where we lack privileges. Our rank unconsciousness no doubt irritates those around us, especially those who have less rank than we do. This tension around rank also makes it difficult to be open about our identities and associated privileges. We have all experienced some level of bullying and social sanctioning, and we can easily fall back on feeling victimized. But when we unilaterally claim victimhood, we marginalize the social oppression of others.

Disaggregating all the aspects of your diverse identities—the history, the pain, and the privilege—creates a basis for more sincere and transparent communication. But to accomplish this, you need to cultivate self-love and generosity. Take care of yourself, but don't automatically expect others to grant you the space for self-love, especially if you are part of a group that has oppressed others.

The checklist below is meant as a guide for creating trusting relationships with your clients and patients so they are better able to follow treatment recommendations. It is an incomplete list of questions that reflect experiences on the social ladder that may relate to your community relationships and health. Remember your loving grandmother, or call on your inner grandmother, and be kind with yourself as you explore the questions below.

Exercise: Desegregating and Disaggregating Information

Disaggregating aspects of your own identity:

- What is your age, sex, gender identity, race, ethnicity, class, religion, sexual orientation, primary language, education level, health status, and legal status?
- Think about a few experiences that have shaped your life.
- How do these attributes of your identity inform your worldview?
- How segregated did you grow up? How segregated is your current life?
- Where do you stand along the spectrum between believing "everyone is the same" and "everyone is different"?
- Where do you stand on the spectrum between believing "I earned my privileges" and "my privileges are based on fortuitous circumstances"?
- What is your relative position on the social status ladder?
- Think of a few adverse events that have changed your life.
- When and how have you experienced discrimination based on race, class, gender, religion, sexual orientation, age, physical ability, size, or other difference?
- How comfortable are you with strong emotions such as anger?
- When you put some effort into a project, how much reward do you experience?
- When were you last thanked or applauded in your family environment? When were you last recognized or promoted at work?
- When did you last feel truly seen?
- How isolated do you feel?
- How much control do you feel you have over your work and home environment?

Disaggregating aspects of a patient's or client's identity:

- What is their age, sex, gender identity, race, ethnicity, religion, class, sexual orientation, primary language, education level, health status, and legal status?
- To the best of your knowledge, what are some of the main experiences that have shaped their life?
- What level of childhood trauma and other adverse events have they experienced? What are some of those events?
- How segregated did they grow up, and how segregated is their current life?
- What is their relative position on the social status ladder?
- When they put some effort into a project or work, how much reward do they experience?
- When were they last thanked or applauded in their family environment? When were they last recognized or promoted at work?
- When did they last feel truly seen?
- How isolated do they feel?
- How much control do they feel they have over their work and home environment?

As I discussed above I embody most demographic attributes associated with centrality and privilege in the community I live in. I am a white, cisgender, heterosexual man who is educated, financially and legally secure, and in good health. My age is slowly bringing me into a group that has some limitations to accessing resources and power. As an immigrant and non-native English speaker, I sometimes feel like an outsider, especially in conversations that include jokes and cultural innuendos that I don't understand because I grew up outside of the United States. When the group discussion is fast and lively, I might feel disadvantaged in my ability to follow the thread of discussion and bring myself in.

As I continue to share my personal history, I am aware that my privileges might be triggering for some readers. My intent is to demonstrate some self-reflection and to inspire readers to think how your history, privileges, and disadvantages have all contributed to make you who you are.

I grew up in a middle-class, French-speaking family that lived in a German-speaking town in Switzerland. My parents had moved from the French-speaking region of the country to Basel, which had more economic and employment opportunities. This made me bilingual and bicultural, and I remember one occasion of being ridiculed by my German teacher in front of my peer classmates. I had written an essay that shared some French cultural values, and this teacher, a sympathizer with Nazi Germany, had used my essay to humiliate me in front of my class. This experience opened my eyes to the reality of cultural dissonances and discrimination. It made me understand what it means to be in a minority position.

I remember spending many vacations in my grandmother's winery estate. We enjoyed the pleasures of playing outside and supporting the farm work by picking cherries, walnuts, and grapes. We were often paired with seasonal workers who came from Algeria and Tunisia. They spoke little French and were very warm and friendly with us. We spent many hours in the dining room beside the kitchen, where they ate their meals. Listening to the foreign sounds, I was intrigued by the differences I started to grasp.

My grandmother had a tradition of drinking her early evening absinthe aperitif in the winter garden of her house. Her friends knew they could drop in then and reminisce about the past. Many of the stories I heard recounted colonial experiences of living in Algeria and Madagascar and managing colonial plantations.

When I was a bit older, my aunt shared how she and my uncle had helped the Algerian FLN, the socialist political party and nationalist movement that fought the war against the French "pieds noirs," or colonialists. Under secrecy and danger, my aunt and uncle had helped the FLN safeguard the treasury of the movement.

As a child, I didn't understand the historical and political contexts of what I was witnessing and surrounded by, but I absorbed the cultural systems and hierarchies that continued to live through my family.

My mother often spoke to me about the Edict of Nantes, signed in 1598 by King Henry IV of France. This edict granted the Calvinist Protestants of France (also known as *Huguenots*) substantial rights in the Catholic nation. In 1685, Louis XIV, the grandson of Henry IV, revoked the edict and declared Protestantism illegal. This led to the religious persecution of Protestants in France and to my ancestors fleeing France at risk of their lives and seeking safety in Switzerland. With this story, my mother imbued me with a Huguenot identity, and I began to understand the reality of persecution and the possibility of becoming a refugee.

After I moved to the United States, my wife gave me a book about the history of the Moors.[57] This book was edited by an African-American historian who, in the pursuit of working on the history of Black slavery, came upon this information. *Moor* is a term that describes North-Saharan and sub-Saharan African Muslims and Arabs who invaded and occupied the Iberian Peninsula for 800 years. The coat of arms of my father's family, Morin, depicts the heads of three Moors.

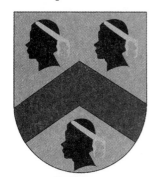

I had long been intrigued by this fact, but I didn't know its significance. Then I read in the history book that many Moors, after they were expelled from Spain in the early 17th century, fled not only back to Africa but also north into France and Germany. I was surprised to find a picture of our family's coat of arms in the book. Thus, I discovered that "Morin" comes from "Moor" and that the Morin coat of arms symbolizes my family's lineage back to Christianized Moors, capturing another complex story of cultural and religious persecution. Through intermarriage, my family's Muslim heritage evolved into the fate and persecution of Protestant Huguenots in France, who fled to Switzerland.

Later, this history intersected with colonialism and revolutionary liberation movements.

This history also exposes the roots of present-day white supremacy and dominance. The heads of the three Moors on my family's coat of arms remind me of war trophies—the slaughter of people of color to maintain racial power. My aunt's support of Algerian freedom fighters was courageous but doesn't let me off the hook for my complicit participation in structures of systemic racism or for the fact that I benefit from white privilege.

Throughout my childhood and early adulthood, race-based difference was a nonexistent topic. All my teachers in elementary and high school were white men, except for one white woman teacher I had in high school. There was one refugee girl from Tibet in my grade school. This trend continued in medical school, where all my professors were white men. So my upbringing was one of financial and educational privilege and a deep-rooted belief in white and male superiority. That didn't make me a bad person, but rather an uninformed and biased person. It also made me tacitly, unfailingly, and unintentionally complicit in perpetuating systemic racism.

In Senegal, as a white medical doctor, I practiced a form of colonial medicine that minimally partnered with the local communities. It wasn't until my doctoral studies, which focused on health psychology, that I woke up to the one-sidedness of my views. For the first time I learned about health disparities caused by systemic oppression. I remember reading that in virtually every area of medicine in the United States, Black patients as a group fare the worst. This shocked me, and I wondered, why is medicine not focused more on addressing this? One reason, I later discovered, is because only around 5 percent of practicing physicians are Black, compared with more than 13 percent of Americans overall.[58] Black patients fare worse because of the inherent bias and prejudice that persists in medicine.

When I was 40, I left Switzerland and emigrated to the United States because I felt too segregated and insulated from the world in my home country. Many people envy my Swiss heritage and don't understand why I would choose to leave its cultural, economic, and geographical privileges behind. Switzerland is seen as this ideal gem of privileges; who would want to emigrate? Obviously, there are many social hierarchies in Switzerland as well; not everything is hunky-dory there either. But for me, in its insularity, Switzerland was too protected from many of the world's issues. Working as a medical doctor in Africa had planted the seed in me that I needed to expose myself to other perspectives and experiences. Emigrating to the United States meant for me that I had to temporarily rescind some of my privileges. I was not able to remain licensed as a medical doctor and was forced to start a new professional career and work my way back up the social status ladder.

I live in a part of Portland that was originally diverse and is becoming more and more gentrified. My workplace, Lutheran Community Services Northwest, is probably the most diverse work environment in Portland. My colleagues and I speak 42 different languages, and most of us are refugees or immigrants. We share diverse cultural, religious, and educational backgrounds and are united by a common passion for assisting and resettling newly arriving refugees. In my association with Process Work, I am exposed to many other areas of diversity, and I have friends who are part of the LBGTQ community.

This bit of personal history is a slice of a much broader smorgasbord of experiences that shape my awareness and my ability to have communal intelligence. As a reader, you might see trends and patterns that I remain blind to. What I can see is that my history has shaped my curiosity about the intersection between individual and community experiences and the relevance of social, cultural, and historical perspectives. I live and have lived a privileged life with all the blind spots and biases that are a natural consequence of such circumstances. I need the help, patience, and goodwill of other people to grow and become more aware. I lived a relatively safe and secure life, and the minor trauma that my German teacher caused me gives me some minimal understanding of what it can mean to be and feel marginalized. I think it gave me an impetus to study the social aspects of health and medicine.

I share these personal stories to stimulate you to look back at your own life and discover the web of patterns and experiences that will shape your unique ability to understand the experiences of your patients, clients, friends, and families. These experiences are the building blocks of your distinct communal intelligence.

Big Medicine and Communal Intelligence

Big Medicine relies on the awareness of Deep Democracy, the multi-layered and multi-phased approach to human experience. Drawing from communal intelligence, Big Medicine addresses the systemic and sociopolitical aspects of health and medicine as well as the less tangible relational and feeling experiences that arise when we encounter these systems. Big Medicine embraces anti-oppression, racial and health equity, and other diversity and inclusion practices by cultivating a deep relationship with our clients and their communities and seeking ongoing feedback from them. To better serve the diverse communities of Portland, we also developed a culturally specific community health worker (CHW) training course. We have been able to train and certify 52 new CHWs who come from eight different countries and speak 12 different languages.

Big Medicine sees the impact of disparities and inequities with candor and sobriety and advocates for change, justice, and liberation. It explores tools and practices that foster understanding of diverse point of views, create commonalities, and facilitate growth, supporting the whole through a spirit of eldership.

Big Medicine advocates for equity and not just equality. Equality stresses equal distribution of and access to resources; for example, *equal* access to health insurance means that everyone has the same right to subsidized healthcare coverage based on income levels. In contrast, *equitable* access to health insurance adds, for example, access to culturally specific services and information translated into minority languages, giving non-English speakers a chance to receive culturally competent services and the necessary information to enroll. On a broader level, we all benefit from equitable strategies.

Here is a trivial example. Many establishments have an equal number of gender-segregated bathroom stalls. But, women take an average of about two minutes longer to use the bathroom, which means they often must wait longer for an empty stall, and their female or male companions also have to wait for them. Equitable numbers of bathroom stalls would mean more stalls in the women's room than the men's, and this would benefit both (or all) genders.

To achieve equal health outcomes—the same opportunity for individuals and communities to stay healthy—we need to foster equitable strategies. Diversity consciousness is a prerequisite for implementing equitable strategies and achieving equal outcomes. Understanding differences in identity, power, rank, opportunity, values, and behaviors is the bedrock for communal intelligence and creating equitable systems, policies, and outcomes. This understanding is at the heart of sustainable relationships and good health.

Big Medicine is about building communal relationships that nurture the best possible conditions for good health. If you want to share a meal with your family and you have a two-year-old child as well as a ten-year-old, if you give each of them a regular chair, they won't be able to participate equally. You need to give the two-year old a high chair for her to have the same opportunity to be part of the family meal. And every family member will benefit from everybody being included in the family activity. If as a provider, you value everybody's well-being, you need to open up to the diversity of lived experiences. Serving an individual who has fewer privileges will require a different approach than serving someone with more majority privileges. We must be aware, though, that when we are in a helping role and working with someone from an underprivileged group, even well-intended interventions can be patronizing. For example, imagine that I, a white man, coach an African-American woman who works in a sexist environment and is suffering from depression, I might be tempted to urge her to fight that sexist behavior and empower herself. However, with that impulse I might be failing to acknowledge her true power, and I know little about the complexity of being a strong woman of color in a white society.

Dr. Damon Tweedy, a Black psychiatrist, recounts in a *New York Times* opinion piece[59] great examples of this important cultural sensitivity:

> Several years ago, for example, I met a recently retired black man who had been referred to me for treatment of depression. He had become increasingly dispirited by the fact that the town where he had raised his children had transformed into a community full of poor schools, single mothers, and young black men in the criminal justice system.
>
> Rather than prescribe him an antidepressant pill, as another doctor had done, I encouraged him to talk in depth about his early life in the 1940s and '50s and the positive influences that had helped him succeed. Discussing his life in this way made him feel more confident about his ability to touch other lives, even though he couldn't fix larger social problems. He helped put together a local program that introduced poor black kids to chess and golf, an endeavor that made him feel better than he had in many years. Periodically, he leaves me messages saying that he is still doing well and thanking me for my help.
>
> Another time, I worked with a young woman who struggled with her biracial identity. Her black father had been abusive to her white mother when she was a child, and she found herself both afraid of and hostile toward black men. Because she physically resembled her father in many ways, she had also turned these negative feelings inward.

Not surprisingly, her initial impression of me was unfavorable, but a friend encouraged her to come back to see me.

Over the next several months, we talked about every aspect of race imaginable, and by the end, she found herself more at peace and better able to see black men as individuals. For the first time, she even met a black man whom she began dating. She no longer felt depressed or severely anxious.

My experience as a patient may also be instructive. I received a diagnosis of high blood pressure as a first-year medical student, and although I knew perfectly well that I needed to change my high-salt, high-fat diet, I just couldn't do it. Of course, it was hard to give up what was familiar and enjoyable. But an equally important part was my resistance to assimilating and adopting behaviors that I associated with well-to-do whites—eating salads and drinking fruit smoothies, for example—even though I knew that this defiance was ultimately self-defeating.

Only after many failed attempts have I been able to consistently do the right thing with my health. Today I take this experience into the exam room. While patients ultimately must take responsibility for their own lives, it is helpful to have a doctor who understands, and doesn't dismiss, behavior patterns that are often rooted in a cultural history.

As members of socially overvalued groups, white people, straight people, and men often believe we know more about oppression than we actually do. We think we have insight into what an African-American woman client is experiencing, when in fact we have no idea at all. Active, courageous deep listening is a more valuable practice in this situation.

But again, the main point is that by addressing our client's diverse needs and supporting her wellness, we benefit as well. This is the true meaning of community health: By addressing the diverse needs of individuals, you serve the community. One well member of the community helps the whole. We are all part of the same community fabric and will feel the consequences of ill health of any of its members.

Developing relationships and building awareness about the differences in lived experiences is at the core of Big Medicine. Big Medicine addresses the systemic need to abolish avoidable health inequities and promote social justice and health justice. It also fosters relationship around diversity to come together and build stronger communities. Big Medicine works for solutions and systemic changes as well as for better relationships and more sustainable communities.

The advocacy we need in order to create more sustainable communities and a better world is embedded in the phase nature of process. Communal intelligence moves through phases that incorporate consensus reality, Dreaming, and essence features. There are times for focusing on ourselves and our own tribe, paying little attention to the larger community (Phase 1). Other times, when issues get polarized, tensions and conflict arise (Phase 2). These tensions can push us until we are forced to open to other points of view, find common ground, and develop greater awareness and eldership (Phase 4). And finally, we can find deep meaning and connection through our sense of belonging to a family, lineage, community, and—when everything else is lacking—to some innate place on earth (Phase 4).

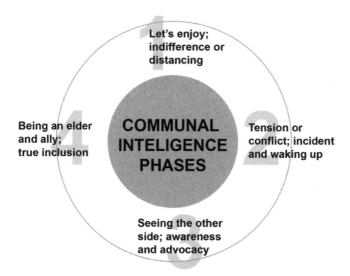

Figure 6. Phases of Communal Intelligence

I want to close this chapter by reflecting back to the situation of the Kitara family. Their medical case managers took the approach that the parents could not get well as long as their daughters back home in Syria remained in danger. They believed that the parents' health symptoms were an expression of their guilt about surviving and their solidarity with their daughters. They are advocating with the UN high commission for refugees and the U.S. government to grant the daughters refugee status on humanitarian grounds. The case managers are practicing courageous listening and holding the tension of facing their limitations to help. As providers, we often face difficult situations that appear hopeless. In Big Medicine, our Phase 4 eldership, allyship, and essence work at times require us to be patient and to support whatever arises, even when it is uncomfortable, and to use our awareness for the overall Process.

Social structures create health benefits for people at the top of the social ladder while making marginalized people sicker. These systems are at the root of the current opioid crisis, the many deaths of Blacks and whites by overdose, the police killings of people of color, the suicide epidemic among transgender and gay people, and the multiple health disparities that marginalized people experience. These social wrongs must be a wake-up call for all of us. They are an opportunity for us to step outside our comfort zone, learn from each other, and create a better world.

Chapter 9

POWER DYNAMICS
AND RELATIONSHIPS

RELATIONSHIPS CAN BE both medicine and poison. They make us sick and help us heal; they nurture our development and cause trauma and suffering; they lift our souls and spirits and crush us into despair and depression.

We are entangled in a complex web of relationships that shape our identities and ways of being in the world. Relationships help us become who we are. They start in the womb as we passively receive our mother's emotional response to her environment. They continue as we learn to mimic our parents' expressions and become aware of our own feelings and other mental states. They help us "optimize" our sense of who we are and who we should be as we learn to conform and fit in the communities we are part of. They create health and wellness, and they contribute to sickness and early death. In terms of Big Medicine, relationships are a source of reflection about our own diversity and our potential for both growth and hurt.

I am part of a care team for Eileen, a white woman with severe and long-lasting gastrointestinal problems. She is unable to eat and drink via her mouth and is fed with the help of tubes that lead directly into her bowel. A central line gives her additional fluids. She has chronic pain from a genetic disorder that affects her joints. These compounded problems mean that she is unable to live a normal life. Medically, her symptoms are inadequately explained, and doctors struggle to make sense of what is happening.

Tibetan Buddhist teacher Chokyi Nyima Rinpoche explains in his book *Medicine & Compassion*[60] that caregivers suffer when their patients fail to respond to their care. That suffering can translate into becoming defensive and blaming the patient. This reaction is exactly what Eileen is experiencing from some of her caregivers. In her youth, Eileen was a ballet dancer, and she fits to some degree the profile of someone with an eating disorder. Eileen rejects this idea and sincerely explains that she never had a difficult relationship with food but that she has developed, over the past two years of not being able to ingest any food, a disordered attitude towards food. This for her is an important difference, in that her disordered attitude is not the cause of but rather a side effect of her symptoms. She feels the prejudice that accompanies the label of "eating disorder." One time, as she was being hospitalized, a doctor yelled at her that she was doing it all to herself.

This type of profiling and abuse is a common experience for people who suffer from chronic conditions that evade medical explanation. What Eileen is experiencing is a form of relational abuse of power and rank. The abuse gets amplified by social dynamics. If it is a male caregiver who is humiliating and shaming a woman patient, it adds extra layers of hurt. Imagine if Eileen were a person of color and the caregiver were white, how much more damaging this interaction would be.

Eileen's story exemplifies the importance of approaching relationships from an individual, personal perspective as well as through a social and structural lens. Besides being traumatized by her body's failings, Eileen also has a personal history of trauma. Her anxiety and reactive depression are adjustments to difficult life circumstances and challenging experiences. In this complex situation, it is difficult to parse what is at the root of what. The search for linear, causal associations with specific cures and treatments is inadequate.

In contrast, Big Medicine's holistic approach is centered on the patient's experience and process. For Eileen, this entails discussing the history of her teenage years (when some of her symptoms started), how she experiences her symptoms, how she and her family have adjusted to managing her chronic symptoms, and how the responses of others have affected her, as well as the support, prejudice, and hurt she has experienced on her journey with chronic illness.

In one of our recent sessions, Eileen explored her experience of pain. She focused on one body part and drew a sketch of her pain experience (see below). Looking at what she drew, she thought of Blenny, an anglerfish character in the movie *Finding Nemo*.

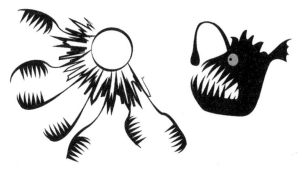

Figure 7. Eileen's Energy Sketch and Blenny from *Finding Nemo*

We found a photograph of Blenny and compared the teeth in her sketch with the teeth of the anglerfish. We brainstormed together about how she is on the receiving end of her pain's burning sharpness (the teeth) as well as of her providers' misuse of power. Then came the question of how she could assimilate the teeth and use them as a protective tool. Naturally, her usual identity is more like that of a smaller fish, one that Blenny would eat. The last thing Eileen wanted was to embrace a quality that causes her both emotional and physical pain. What a dilemma! Together we brainstormed about how she could use her "teeth" and strength in a way that would be acceptable to her.

In this chapter, I will discuss what science can bring to understanding relationships, how relationships impact our bodies, and how we get socialized into structures that contribute to health disparities.

I will examine the importance of power and rank dynamics in provider-client relationships and explore racism as an example of systemic oppression that is one of the root causes for health disparities. As we can see from Eileen's story, Big Medicine recognizes all these contributing factors and looks for answers beyond the trauma.

What Science Brings to Relationships

Modern neurobiology helps explain how we respond to each other emotionally and physically. Big Medicine combines these findings with Process-informed coaching methods to facilitate relationships and ease their impacts on our bodies.

Let's start with some relevant theories. Interpersonal neurobiology, a new interdisciplinary field developed by Daniel Siegel and Allan Schore, is based on the theory that we are who we are as individuals by way of our relationships to one another. We are social beings, and it turns out that our brains are—via their stress hormones, mirror neurons, and epigenetics—constantly reshaping themselves based on our relationship experiences. Neuroimaging studies have shown that by altering the activity and structure of the connection between neurons, experiences are able to shape our memory, emotion, and self-awareness.[61] For example, we've all had the experience that when we are stressed out, our memory works differently. And when we let ourselves relax and daydream, new ideas emerge.

Also interesting is the fact that emotional and physical pain are processed in the same regions of the brain, perhaps because both forms of pain challenge our survival. Through neurotransmitters, both forms of pain trigger similar cascades of physiological changes in our bodies, and they can both be treated by the same type of drugs (i.e., Tylenol or acetaminophen)[62] or the same type of psychological interventions (i.e., mindfulness-based stress reduction).[63] Likewise, neurofeedback, meditation, mindfulness, and psychotherapy help alleviate both emotional pain (anxiety and depression) and physical pain. And, because our relationships, emotions, brain and body are so intertwined, practices that address physical pain have emotional benefits, and therapies that address emotional ailments have physical benefits.

For Siegel, *presence*, which he defines as a "state of attunement, resonance, and trust," is one of the most powerful forces that foster natural healing. He views presence as a quality that is central to relationships. As both an internal and interpersonal process, presence is the internal awareness that enables us to take in what is emerging moment by moment—and it is the interpersonal attunement that honors people for their differences and allows for healthy, supportive relationships.[64] Presence is also a mental state that offers impressive physical effects, such as improving epigenetic regulation (see below) and increasing telomerase, an enzyme that counteracts some cellular aging mechanisms. Siegel asserts that presence, as a healing quality, can be strengthened through secure attachment, mindfulness meditation, and effective psychotherapy. Cultivating presence promotes effective therapy and healing, he says.[65]

Mirror neurons[66] play an important role in modulating our relationships. These specialized nerve cells are active both when we engage in a certain activity as well as when we observe another person performing the same activity. For example, mirror neurons fire the same way whether we are grabbing an apple or watching someone else pick up an apple. They allow us to recognize and feel other people's feelings, dissolving the border between ourselves and others. They are a hardwired system that helps us perceive the mind-state of another person and learn to empathize with them. Siegel writes that mirror neurons "automatically and spontaneously pick up information about the intentions and feelings of those around us, creating emotional resonance and behavioral imitation as they connect our internal state with those around us, even without the participation of our conscious mind."[67]

They are also the physiological foundation for developing a sense of personhood and identity. We enact our own self by internally mirroring people around us. The neuroscientist Vilayanur S. Ramachandran has suggested that mirror neurons are central to our self-awareness. Mirror neurons enable us to see another's viewpoint. In addition, mirror neurons facilitate "looking at myself as if someone else is looking at me." Thus, the mirror neurons "that originally evolved to help you adopt another's point of view [are] turned inward to look at your own self."[68] Mirror neurons help us construct a neural map of being simultaneously an "I" and part of an interdependent "us."

Our brains communicate with one another, constantly picking up signals and information and processing the exchange in ways that can be detrimental or uplifting. Neurobiology gives us knowledge of the mechanism of these interactions and hints at healthy and healing pathways, such as the benefits of certain relational attitudes and behaviors (i.e., presence).

Like much of all science and medicine, neurobiology tends to be linear, causal, and dualistic in its approach. Big Medicine, in turn, with its Process-informed perspective, sees the importance of understanding science-based insights as well as recognizing the more cyclical and holistic path of nature. Conflict and trauma are to be prevented, and they are also integral components of a cycle of life that goes through phases, one of which is more discordant. Presence, then, includes a sense of eldership that is attuned to the fact that conflict and tension are natural occurrences with purpose and meaning, and they need not be thwarted prematurely. Peace, harmony, trust, and resonance are not desired end states but stages in an ever-evolving cyclical process.

The Role of Genes

As humans, we share 99.5 percent of our genome or genetic makeup. We differ in only 0.5 percent of our genes. Our genetic pool, the biological basis of who we are, changes very slowly over time from one generation to another when a mutation becomes advantageous and significant in an evolutionary sense. The expression and utilization of genes, the way they pattern proteins, is more vulnerable to environmental influences. Stress hormones and other factors can turn a gene on and off and influence the output of genes.

This outside impact on the operation of our genes is called *epigenetics*. This discipline helps us understand both the possible positive and detrimental impact of environmental and relational factors. Micro-aggressions, abuse, and trauma have negative physiological impacts that start prior to our conception and birth. On the other hand, supportive relationships and stimulating experiences have beneficial influences that can repair the damages done.

In other words, while we all share the same genetic makeup or basic notes, we differ in how we play the notes and what tunes we compose with the notes we play (epigenetics). These tunes are strongly influenced by our personal and family histories and the social environment we live in.

We are embedded in a surrounding world of relationships and community interactions that significantly affect us and determine the course and outcome of aspects of our lives.[69] These exchanges are based on signals (both verbal and non-verbal) and actions. They can be rooted in structures and systems that carry implicit information and meaning.

The Role of Power

States of power, privilege, and rank stratify our society, transmitting signals to its members from support to hostility to neglect. Rank and power are composed of various elements. Rank can be situational or contextual (often referred to as *status*). It works on the individual level and on the systemic level (that is, the rank of a certain subgroup of people). On the individual level, rank has social, psychological, and spiritual aspects. I will discuss all these types below.

We are familiar with status differences, that is, the social stratification of power and rank based on financial resources, education, race, gender, sexual orientation, and other factors. Certain social classifications and groups are imbued with legal, political, economic, and social rights and privileges, while other groups are denied the same. Groups are also granted or denied access to tangible and intangible resources, such as self-worth, visibility, positive expectations, emotional and psychological self-determination, freedom of movement, the sense of belonging, and a sense of entitlement to all the above.

The repetitive experiences we are exposed to in our interactions with each other and within our social environments socialize us into our unique status of social power and rank. This process of socialization generates and maintains thoughts, perceptions, opinions, and actions.[70] Social powers are also embedded in institutional systems and sociopolitical structures. They impact housing segregation, health disparities, the content of history and geography books, voting rights, disability accommodations, and much more.

We are more accustomed to recognizing status and less accustomed to recognizing the psychological rank and power we develop as we confront and experience adversity or other challenges. Overcoming health problems and other difficulties can lead to a greater sense of resilience and agency (see below). This can translate into personal power, charisma, and leadership abilities.

Individual spiritual rank is a strength we draw from our connection to a transpersonal source of power, be it Nature, God, the Goddess, or other divine presence. In terms of the phases, gaining access to Phase 4 —which comprises a sense of detachment, a wide perspective, eldership, and connection to our essence and true self—often gives us charisma and power.

Rank is also contextual. Certain outer situations grant us momentary access to feeling more empowered even when we may feel socially disempowered. A typical example is being in a helper or teaching position, such as a counselor, doctor, nurse, caregiver, coach, or instructor.

Or compare the ranks of a teacher and a principal, a bank teller and a customer, a custodian and a receptionist. The rank we hold in a particular context—how we perceive ourselves and are perceived by others—shifts with the context. A school librarian has a lot of power in her library room, where she is in control. When she comes to speak to the school principal, she has less power. The power lines shift with the context. But they are still influenced by social categories. The school custodian, for example, is more likely to be a male and, in certain social environments, a person of color. The librarian, in turn, is probably a white female.

Next, it is important to remember that all these layers of ranks intersect. A white woman may focus on her low rank as a woman and marginalize her high rank as a white person. Each person's privileges stack up in a different way. Typically, we are far more aware of someone else's higher rank in comparison to us than we are of our own higher ranks and privileges.

Normal health and physical ability are their own sets of rank and privileges. Diseases and disabilities are at times apparent but are frequently hidden. Years ago, I coached Julie, who had a brain injury that caused a seizure disorder. Her pre-injury identity was of being extroverted and highly efficient in multi-tasking and completing professional and social tasks. Since her stroke, she experienced herself as being slower and more confused. To others, she outwardly appeared as her old normal self; they didn't understand the changes she was undergoing. Her husband distanced himself from her, unable to let go of his old standards and expectations of their relationship. Julie acutely suffered from the loss of status and power she endured.

Social and relational settings come with both explicit and unwritten rules. Certain behaviors and ways of being are socialized into us, and we internalize these social and relationship patterns. When Julie was thrown out of her old position, she had to navigate a sense of loss, emotional unsteadiness, and stress from the interruption to her familiar patterns of life.

Her injury had an added side effect: She became more emotional. Tears would well up all the time. They embarrassed her, as she often experienced them as inopportune and misplaced. Over time, she became more comfortable with them and was able to turn them into a source of strength and psychological power.

As health professionals, we practice in environments where all these social forces and patterns interplay. We carry our own internalized and unconscious biases, rank-based experiences, and social rules. We embody our social ranks (and lack thereof), as well as the contextual ranks we are granted by our profession. We are influenced by our personal histories and social wounds and the learnings we've been able to gain. We serve individuals and communities that come to us with their own histories and socially patterned experiences and behaviors. A good first step toward greater awareness of rank dynamics is to learn how to use our own powers.

Exercise: Learn to Know and Use Your Powers

1. Identify all the ranks and powers that you hold (social, psychological, spiritual, contextual). Make notes about these.

2. What mainstream idea(s) do you sometimes use to discriminate against yourself? For example: Do you use your age, appearance, health, size, skin color, gender, or sexual orientation to put yourself down? How do you counter these thoughts?

3. What personal powers and inner resources do you draw on to get out of bed in the morning, to get by each day, to overcome challenges, to remain creative, to give your life a sense of direction and purpose?

4. A dream-level form of personal power can be associated with early childhood night dreams or memories. In early childhood, we are less influenced by social patterns, so these memories and dreams bring forth some innate schemes. Recall the weirdest, scariest, strangest figure from an early childhood dream or

memory. Explore what its energy feels like and express it in a gesture or sketch. Give that energy a name and ponder how you can use it as one of your personal powers.

As a white, straight, educated, and financially secure man, I hold many social powers and privileges. But occasionally I find myself thinking that at my age of 61, I should stop doing certain things. Just recently, I caught myself thinking that, because of being near the "end" of my career, I should not apply to participate in an intensive social action training. I had to convince myself that I deserved a spot. Also, when I experience a health problem, I sometimes think that as a health-conscious physician, I should be better than that. I judge myself for being sick and not staying healthy. I am fortunate to have a partner and friends with whom I can share these thoughts and process them.

Over the years I have learned and have been supported to become more compassionate toward myself. This has allowed me to follow my passion of thinking deeply about medicine, and the more I do this, the more I am inspired by the creative process that directs my life. There is something bigger than me that reveals itself in my night dreams and in the thoughts that pop up in the middle of the night.

In my childhood dream, I am waking up because our apartment is on fire. I escape to the second-floor landing of the apartment, and as I start to run down the stairs, two black panthers are climbing the stairs from below. When I unfold the energy of the panthers, I come up with a slow-moving, centered, and looming power. It is present and available but remains dormant when not challenged. Panthers, in my imagination, are also shy and live hidden in the jungle. Over the years I have learned to appreciate aspects of this panther power in myself. I can see it in my steadfast pursuit of social and health justice.

Atul Gawande, a surgeon and staff writer for the *New Yorker,* writes:

> Much of society has become like an airplane boarding line,
> with different rights and privileges for zones one to ninety-
> seven, depending on your wealth, frequent-flier miles, credit
> rating, and S.A.T. scores; and many of those in line think
> —though no one likes to admit it—that they deserve what
> they have more than the others behind them. ... Regarding
> people as having lives of equal worth means recognizing
> each as having a common core of humanity. Without being
> open to their humanity, it is impossible to provide good care
> to people... To see their humanity, you must put yourself in
> their shoes. That requires a willingness to ask people what
> it's like in those shoes. It requires curiosity about others and
> the world beyond your boarding zone."[71]

We believe we are individuals, independent of each other—but we are
firmly embedded in a web of powerful rank- and power-based social
patterns. These have direct emotional and physiological effects that we
pass onto future generations.

Personal powers are embedded in a context of social arrangements.
Our membership in social groups and the larger social dynamics between these groups have important health consequences. In the next
few pages, I will explore intergroup power dynamics, health-related
biases and stigmas, our tendency to remain in the comfort of our in-
groups, and racism as an example of oppression and cause of health
disparities. The individual and collective use of power creates and
destroys health.

The Role of Love, Abuse, and Microaggressions

The Grant Study, a study of 268 men over a period of 75 years, showed that sustained, warm, intimate relationships predicted emotional and physical well-being. Love, the study's main researcher says, was the main source of the men's happiness and wellness. This study of adult development revealed how beneficial positive and nurturing social connections are to health and well-being. In contrast, the Kaiser Permanente Adverse Childhood Experiences Study proved that abuse, neglect, and microaggressions have serious damaging health impacts. And the Whitehall studies of British civil servants described the link between social status and health and how the experience of low rank led to negative health outcomes.[72]

All these studies have one thing in common: they demonstrate how important relationships are for health, both in a positive and negative sense. Though we know how important love is for well-being, the experience of love is a privilege that is granted to some more than others because of a multitude of family and social factors. The important point here is that our particular family and social arrangements enable some to be more generous and loving while forcing others into abuse, neglect, and survival mode. This is why our sense of the empowerment, privilege, and rank (of both ourselves and our communities) is so relevant to relationships, and to how relationships impact our physical and emotional wellness.

When people are sick, the social marginalization of illness adds another layer of harm. The denial of illness as a natural process makes sick people feel ashamed and guilty. Not being able to remain healthy comes with a form of implicit blame. As an example, Eileen's lived experience of her illness is complex. She feels traumatized by outer experiences and by her body. She senses the helplessness of her providers and their indirect criticism. Her depression and hopelessness are a natural response to her dire circumstances and these hurtful relational dynamics.

In a recent group session, I helped facilitate the Process of Robert, a client who was in physical pain from a resurging chronic disease process. But his main distress was about having failed to contain his disease, despite having done everything right. He was in an abusive fight with himself. I helped him take a step back and observe a role-play of his internal conflict. With that detachment, he was able to access an inner elder that expressed compassion for both conflicting sides.

Health Bias and Disease Stigma

Our implicit biases towards health and the stigmatizing of disease are perhaps most rampant around the issue of body size and obesity. Overweight people experience more than their share of shame and blame. Obesity, they are told by their doctor, their loved ones, and the community at large, is a personal failing, an individual character problem. Fat-shaming and bullying is visible and invisible, public and private, hidden and everywhere at the same time. This, even though we know that obesity is predominantly a systemic problem due to poverty, limited access to low-cost healthy foods, a sedentary lifestyle, and industrial systems that promote sugary and processed foods.

As the number of obese individuals has risen, the biases against them have become more severe. More than 40 percent of Americans classified as obese now say they experience stigma on a daily basis, a rate far higher than that reported by any other minority group.[73] And this has a terrible impact on their bodies. According to a 2015 study, fat people who feel discriminated against have shorter life expectancies than fat people who don't. "These findings suggest the possibility that the stigma associated with being overweight," the study concluded, "is more harmful than actually being overweight."[74]

What is true from an epidemiological or public health perspective—namely, the clear link between stigma, trauma, suffering, and negative health outcomes—is more complex on an individual level.

Trauma unfailingly brings suffering in its wake. But suffering can also make us who we are, and we can learn to transform trauma into emotional strength. *Resilience* is the human capacity to turn misfortune into an experience that enhances our quality of life. The impact of adverse fateful events and harmful social arrangements can stimulate, on an individual level, life-affirming forces that foster our sense of purpose and resolve. We use our resilience to promote meaningful change of what originally caused the pain. In Eileen's instance, we can imagine that at some point she will be able to use the power of the pain (the teeth) to advance her understanding of her chronic illness and chronic pain.

What does this mean? It means that we all have more in common than we usually think (It also means that a social construct such as race is biologically meaningless). It also suggests that how we relate to each other and the social arrangements we develop together have a strong impact on how well our bodies and our genes work. This, in turn, affects the course of our physical lives. We are essentially all the same, yet how we treat each other individually and systemically has a huge impact. Our diversity comes from the minimal difference in our genes and, more significantly, from how the genes we all share are expressed. But besides bringing beauty and variety, this diversity leads to jealousy, competition, and wars. It is also used by certain social groups (i.e., white men) to marginalize others and preserve their own privileges and powers.

Considering the very real social disparities and the trauma caused by these disparities, talking about common ground can be inflammatory. But on the other hand, rejecting our shared essence may contribute to perpetuating these disparities.

Tribalism Versus Diversity

To protect ourselves emotionally and psychologically from the impact of dysfunctional social dynamics, we most often adhere to a form of tribalism, remaining more open to some groups of people than others. We build relationships where we feel comfortable, favoring like-minded people over those with different views, beliefs, and values. We shield our individual identity from being challenged by differences and diversity. We critically reject unknown traits and behaviors and conflict with whoever opposes our views. This all makes sense because it helps us feel empowered and more secure of who we are.

On the other hand, this tribalism can make us disregard our own inner diversity and stay closed to potential developmental opportunities. In our night dreams, we embody diverse traits and behaviors and then feel relieved when we wake up and can return to our "normal" selves. Later during the day, we don't realize that we are gossiping about others who are engaged in the behaviors we just dreamed about. We externalize and project the inner diversity we reject in ourselves onto others to stay in our comfort zone.

Another protective mechanism and form of tribalism is *white fragility*, a term coined by Dr. Robin DiAngelo, a white social justice educator. She writes:

> White people in North America live in a social environment
> that protects and insulates them from race-based stress.
> This insulated environment of racial protection builds white
> expectations for racial comfort while at the same time
> lowering the ability to tolerate racial stress, leading to what
> I refer to as White Fragility. White Fragility is a state in which
> even a minimum amount of racial stress becomes intolerable,
> triggering a range of defensive moves. These moves include
> the outward display of emotions such as anger, fear, and
> guilt, and behaviors such as argumentation, silence, and

leaving the stress-inducing situation. These behaviors, in turn, function to reinstate white racial equilibrium.[75]

White people's cognitive biases, our attachment to the comfort of our in-group, and our defensiveness vis-à-vis challenges to our misuse of power all serve to protect our individual and cultural identities. But these behaviors oppress others and create health disparities. They are a form of intellectual and cognitive tribalism.

Psychologist Dan Kahan showed that the more challenged our views are, the more we defend them, and the more dogmatic and closed-minded we become. He framed this as an intellectual form of "circle the wagons, we're under attack" tribal unity: "If you are not with me, you are my enemy."[76] We create a sense of community based on differentiating ourselves from others. Author Brené Brown, in turn, calls the creation of a common enemy a form of "intimacy": Our connection is built on saying bad things about other people, and the intimacy we share is formed on hating the same people.[77]

On an important side note for our current times, cultural psychologist Michele Gelfand explores how we rely on more authoritarian approaches and powerful leaders when we are under threat and higher stress.[78] She confirms what author Karen Stenner has written about perceived threats to the moral order pushing people to endorse authoritarian leaders.[79]

Weaponizing Inclusive Language

Within this tribal mentality, some use political correctness and inclusive language as a coercive moral standard, turning them into weapons of shame. Rightful civility then can become weaponized as a tool to put others down for their lack of racial awareness, cultural competence, and diversity consciousness. What is meant as an anti-oppressive standpoint becomes oppressive in its own right.

The confusion stems from a misunderstanding of the definition of *racism*. If we define racism as an individual, conscious, immoral act, and we are called out for being racist, then shame and defensiveness are a logical response. In this good versus bad individual binary, one cannot be both a good moral person and be complicit with racism.

But racism, as I will explain more in detail later, is much more than individual prejudice. It is the entrenchment of racial prejudices in social narratives, structures, and policies. In this context, unconscious white biases will keep perpetuating. They are salient in their impact and in the way they reinforce collective narratives. We need each other to become more aware of our biases and how they impact people of color and other marginalized groups. But we need to get out of the good/bad binary and the shaming/defensiveness dynamic to address the important forms of systemic oppression.

As Atul Gawande[80] puts it, white people live in a different boarding zone and seating class. As whites, we lead segregated lives, and we think of ourselves as individuals as opposed to members of a group. We receive constant messages that whiteness is valuable and that we deserve the comfort and privileges we were born into. We feel entitled to our comfort, and when we get exposed to racial and social injustice, we don't know how to talk about it. From this standpoint, using politically correct language, while relevant when it is meant to be inclusive, can become a token behavior protecting us from taking a real look at social dynamics and injustices.

Two Basic Questions

I keep coming back to two questions: How can we reconcile our urgent need to abolish systemic oppression and the suffering it creates while also advocating for a relational and facilitative approach that wants to hear *all* voices? And how can we acknowledge the experience of white fragility on one side as well as the reaction of shaming and righteousness on the other side?

Let's return to defining racism. I like the way Ijeoma Oluo explains it: "Prejudice against someone based on race, when those are simultaneously reinforced by systems of power."[81] Robin DiAngelo writes, "When a racial group's collective prejudice is backed by the power of legal authority and institutional control, it is transformed into racism, a far-reaching system that functions independently from the intention or self-images of individual actors."[82] These definitions imply that you don't have to be "a racist" to be part of a racist system or to say and do things that are unconscious expressions of that racist system and its conditionings. This form of racism is not about an individual's conscious intolerance. Individual behavior is relevant only in the sense of how it reinforces racial stereotypes and supports the unjust distribution and use of power. And it impacts oppressed people's health, as Dr. Roberto Montenegro says in an NPR podcast about microaggressions and health. The day he got his Ph.D., Dr. Montenegro was mistaken for a valet at the symphony. He turned red and his heart was pounding. Those were signs that his body was feeling acutely stressed.[83]

Individual racism also exists, of course. Along with misogyny, homophobia, and other forms of bigotry, individual racism is harmful and needs to be rectified. But more importantly, it supports and reinforces a system of power that uses the same prejudices to discriminate against whole groups of people and preserve the power for wealthy straight white men.

Oluo's definition of racism also implies that we cannot fix racially based systemic injustices on an emotional or relational basis alone—an overhaul of our institutions is needed. When as white people we prioritize our individual needs through our defensiveness and ignore the reality of structural oppression and the institutional support of racial bias, we perpetuate racism. Every voice is important; every experience is valuable. The question we must ask ourselves is: Do our experiences impact our chances of being treated fairly and humanely, of receiving services, of accessing economic opportunities? Therein lies the difference. Others, such as people of color, LGBTQ people, etc. are exposed to greater risks and injustices than straight white people.

When we talk about racism and raise awareness about the consequences of individual behaviors, we need to comment on the systemic impact they have and how they reinforce and participate in unfair collective structures. We need to keep in mind that the issue is not only us but also the system of racism that reveals itself in our statements and actions. We need to remember that although it is important to focus on the individual level, we may risk ignoring the systemic issues and therefore reinforce the existing power structures.

One facilitative approach, in relationship and group work, is to point to the momentary high rank that a person might have in a specific interaction, even though she might identify as a marginalized person. People can gain this psychological rank, paradoxically, through overcoming hardship and advocating for change. This intervention can bring awareness to the momentary power dynamics and can help resolve conflicts by balancing the overall rank structure. However, if we neglect to mention that the systemic lack of power persists and is unchanged by the individual interaction and resolution, we perpetuate structural racism.

A true relational and facilitative approach to systemic oppression based on race, gender, sexual orientation, and health status will address the momentary complex rank differences while also remembering the structural and historical aspects of oppression—how they impact the relationship and are ongoing outside of the individual relationship scene. The Deep Democracy approach values all voices and differentiates between the many levels and experiences of rank. It also recognizes the blinders that come with privilege and higher rank. It acknowledges that, while there are valid points of view and experiences on all sides, the reality of structural oppression means that the way people of different races, genders, etc. experience society is starkly different. Attempting to equalize experiences that are not equal contributes to ongoing structural oppression. "All Lives Matter": Yes, of course, and no—because humanity isn't systematically stripped from all lives the way it has been, and still is, stripped from the lives of Black people.

Big Medicine recognizes systemic oppression and intergroup power dynamics as social determinants of health. To achieve more equitable access to resources and improved population health, we must address injustices caused by poverty, racism, sexism, healthism, and homophobia. We must support actions at all levels (consensus reality, Dreaming, and essence) to ensure Big Health.

Our common ground and inescapable humanness are important. I understand that if you are in a marginalized place, you might not want to think about this at all. But when we can deeply feel into our commonness, it allows us to relate to diverse human experiences and acknowledge our limitations, blinders, differences, and vulnerabilities. When, in contrast, we stress our differences and criticize the qualities, traits, and behaviors we see in others, we may miss the moments when we engage in them ourselves. Remember, we are all much more aware of other people's rank and abuse of power than we are aware of how we use our own rank and privileges.

The basic truth is that humans are essentially all made of the same material, but our society is structured by social arrangements and rank differences that have huge and deadly impacts. Holding this tension is difficult and not always possible. We must celebrate diversity and fight injustice; and some of us may be able to remember occasionally that we share 99.5 percent of our basic makeup.

Like individual trauma, collective pain brings us suffering and grief. Structural racism and oppression cause damage. But when we can come together in community, and share the pain and learning, we can remind ourselves that we are not alone in our darkness and that we are connected in our pain. This, at times, can lead to powerful change. Brené Brown calls this "the ministry of Presence."[84]

She cites John O'Donohue: "Only holiness will call people to listen now. And the work of holiness is not about perfection or niceness; it is about belonging, that sense of being in the Presence and through the quality of that belonging, the mild magnetic of implicating others in the Presence... This is not about forging a relationship with a distant God but about the realization that we are already within God."[85]

Chapter 10

"I AM": WHO AM I?

LONG AFTER FINISHING medical school, I kept having a recurring nightmare that, although I had passed my medical exams and was practicing medicine, I had to go back to medical school and retake my exams. In the dreams I had a dual identity of being a student of medicine and a practicing doctor. Just recently, that dream took a new turn. I dreamed that I passed my second medical exams and as a graduation gift I received an old leather satchel, one that you could carry on a horse. This bag contained basic woodworking tools.

Over the years, my professional identity has perplexed me. When I was practicing as a medical doctor, even though I achieved recognition as an assistant medical director of a groundbreaking rehabilitation hospital, I often felt like an impostor, one who never truly mastered the knowledge and skills. Then I left medicine, dove into psychology, and started working with people as a coach and counselor. In that role, I carried with me my knowledge of the body and medicine and often got asked to guide my clients on their medical and symptom experience journeys. In my Process Work practice, I have also explored people's experiences with diseases and illnesses.

My recurring dreams about medical school capture my ambivalence and need for more "schooling" and "training," whatever that means in a Dreaming sense. My exploration of Big Medicine and process-oriented psychology brought things together. The disparate fields of medicine and psychology became one, and I was able to metaphorically retake my exams and develop a more congruent identity. My dream graduation present of basic hand tools gives me a direction for my craft. In my mind, it tells me to follow elemental Process steps. With Process, I can see the whole and unify medicine, psychology, and social science.

What intelligence in me has that knowledge and can represent the inner struggles and identity formation in my dream? Who or what is the Dreaming self that knows? Where does that knowing belong?

As I have said, there is a Dreaming intelligence and Process that surpasses our everyday consciousness. This "Dreammaker" and Process Mind is the organizing principle. Over the ages, humans have given it many names: Nature, God, Ubuntu, the Self.

In this chapter, I want to explore the experience of Process Mind through a special inner work practice that Arnold Mindell calls "space-time Dreaming." I want to frame that process in the context of other spiritual and psychological traditions. Space-time Dreaming gives you the experience of being moved. This practice is one way to connect with the manifestation of Process Mind and bridge the paradigmatic gap between inner experiences and outer observations, body and mind, science and psyche. This inner work allows you to explore tensions, conflicts, and unwelcome body experiences; identify the various roles and polarities; and then find some distance from the problems.

This practice will give you insights into what organizes your own conflicted energies and how you can best approach your internal challenges. Its primary goals are not healing and well-being, but rather awareness with and connection to the organizing Process Mind, which gives you some ease but, more importantly, more understanding and meaning. Wellness is more like a beneficial side effect than the goal.

Throughout this chapter, I will explore space-time Dreaming and Process Mind in the context of spiritual traditions and neuroscience. It's a complex underpinning that I won't be able to fully articulate. I apologize in advance to readers who are more spiritually or scientifically inclined than me. I grew up in an environment of institutionalized Christian religion and can't any more embrace many of its concepts and ideas. I am also trained in modern sciences and hold many of their premises to be true, but I feel something is missing. I miss a sense of home in matters of spirit. In that, I am probably not alone; I assume many of my readers might feel the same way. So, what follows is an inquiry and quest. It is fragmented, flawed, and incomplete. It is a beginning.

The tension is between a scientific and material view of the world that is based on data from experiments, and a view of the world that is more based on internal and personal experiences. These inner experiences (see also Chapters 5 and 7), such as the knowing that I experience from my night dreams, cannot be measured or proven. They belong to a world that is intangible and spiritual. Big Medicine is committed to all of it: the physical world as well as to the world of absolutes that transcends the physical body and connects us with spirit, God, Tao, Process Mind, and the Dreammaker.

"I am" is the title that the God of Christians and Jews gave himself in Exodus 3:14 when he reportedly told Moses "I am who I am." Jesus, when he was challenged by the Pharisees, later echoed that wording when he said: "Truly, truly! I say to you, before Abraham was, I am" (John 8: 56-58). Other world religions use similar terminology to describe a Supreme Being. In other words, one can interpret "I am" as a call to become present to yourself and your Process—to unlock your Process Mind. Many traditions help us develop a language and practice for this remembrance. For Big Medicine, this practice of connecting with our Process Mind is the source of our holistic self-healing power, which paradoxically includes illness, disease, and death.

Self in Psychology

"I am," the experience of Self from a psychological vantage point, is an experiential process that is constantly changing. It includes both the self as an object—Me, my hands, my face in the mirror—as well as the self as subject or "I," the one who is seeing the hands or face.

Then, as we interact with the environment, we develop individual and social consciousness and awareness. We use it to differentiate ourselves and to integrate aspects of our experiences into a sense of "I" or "Me"; we enact a Self. Additionally, we have an embodied self, which is the experience of having a particular body; there is a perceiving self who experiences the world from a first-person point of view; there is an agent self who acts in the world; there is an experience of being a continuous and distinctive person over time with a particular story; and there is a social self who responds to feedback from others.

But what is this "I" that combines all these experiences? What organizes us into a coherent Self or "I," and what organizes nature and the universe? The answer, so far, has escaped scientific explanation. Some scientists reduce nature and consciousness to evolution that started with the Big Bang. They reject the notion of intelligent design, explaining consciousness as an emerging faculty that is fully based on the competencies of the lower-level building blocks, i.e., the nerve cells and biological structures that form the brain. They believe that mind, soul, and subjective experiences are, or will be, fully explainable in biological and evolutionary terms.

What Is Consciousness?

It is true that many lower-level biological systems, such as nerve cells, have competence without comprehension or awareness. They respond to information and feedback and adjust their functions competently, even though they don't understand the why and what for. From the point of view of evolutionary biology, comprehension and consciousness appear at an evolutionary step as beneficial side effects. Consciousness, or mind, is a brain function that evolved and survived because of its utility. We can't understand how it works, but that is only a matter of time, scientists believe.

In *Health in Sickness, Sickness in Health,*[86] I used the analogy of a child learning the mechanics of a battery-powered radio as a way to emphasize the gap between brain and mind. In this comparison, the child is not able to fathom where the music comes from and what makes hearing it a pleasurable experience. Knowledge of the outer world—grasping the mechanics of physics and biology—doesn't give us insight into our inner experiences.

Similarly, our knowledge of psychology, our awareness of the role of our family upbringing, our personal history, the mechanics of our thought patterns and stress reactions—these all give us a map of who we are. But, just as a map of New York is not New York, our ideas about ourselves are not who we are. So, who are we? What is the Self? Can you ever know or remember who you are?

How does consciousness happen? Somehow, within our brains, the combined activity of billions of neurons—each one a tiny biological machine—is generating conscious experience. We experience ourselves and our environment through sense-, brain-, and body-mediated mental and interactional processes, many of which remain below the surface of our awareness. The brain doesn't see, taste, feel, or hear the world. It receives electrical impulses from our sensory organs and constructs an experience based on prior learning and expectations, in a process that the neuroscientist Anil Seth[87] calls "controlled hallucinations."[88]

These processes don't reflect outer reality—they are constructed inner experiences that match prior experiences and create coherence. For that purpose, the brain will manipulate the sensory information and create these controlled hallucinations, as long as they make sense. The brain constantly makes best guesses about the source and meaning of the sensory information it receives, and it interprets that information based on context, prior knowledge, and expectations. In essence, we actively generate the world from the inside out.

The same is true for the conscious experience of being a self as a distinct holistic entity. As I have said, there are many ways we experience the self: through our first-person journey in the world, through intention and action, through the coherent personal and social narrative that we develop over time, and through having and being a body.

The experience of being a distinct holistic entity, the lead character in our inner movie, starts with experiencing our bodies from the inside. The sensory information from our internal physiological milieu forms the basis for a primary material "me." Our brains also construct what makes most sense from moment to moment, comparing our expectations with sensory information from the body's inside. We consciously experience what we expect based on past experiences, rather than what violates our expectations.[89] In this way, we predict ourselves into existence, constructing a coherent inner and outer world in a form of controlled hallucinations. Moment by moment, 100 percent of our experience of the world outside is created inside. We experience a model of the world that is optimized for the sensory abilities we have developed as humans. And then, with others, we engage in a social or communal sense making and agreement process to co-create what we call "reality" (see Chapter 4).

Awareness in a Social Context

Our brains and nerve cells don't passively receive information. An organ of relation, the brain interacts with other parts of the body and the world in an ongoing meaning-making process. Consciousness, as we have seen, is an active and creative process. Awareness is also inherently interactional and relational, as it is embedded in a body that interacts with the world and actively creates sense.

Our responses to the environment, our emotions, arise from perceptions of changes in our body. Through physical experiences, the body creates emotions. As William James famously stated, "I don't sing because I am happy; I'm happy because I sing." To prove this, researchers inhibited forehead wrinkling and frowns with botulinum toxin (Botox) and found that their research subjects felt less sad and depressed.[90] If you make someone smile by giving them a pen to hold in their mouth, they feel happier. Our bodies carry us to who we are and how we perceive and experience the world around us. Consciousness is not something that happens passively in an individual brain bubble. It is an active and interactional process between our embodied selves and the world around us.

Compassion, Empathy, Mirroring, and Consciousness

Consciousness, the process of experiencing, is mediated by the body and embedded in the world. It is also basic to the nature of sentient beings. Our feeling responses motivate our actions and choices. As helpers, healers, and providers, one basic motivational feeling we share is compassion. Compassion is an attitude, a way of approaching our needs and the needs of others. It has little to do with whether you consider yourself spiritual or not. From a Buddhist perspective, it is an intrinsic quality that is inherently present in the mind of every person and that we can learn how to access.

Empathy is feeling with someone else. This feeling into someone else's emotions happens through mirroring, the subconscious mimicking of another's nonverbal signals. The act of mirroring activates mirror neurons (discussed in Chapter 9). Mirroring plays an important role in the development of an infant's notion of self. And when we inhibit someone's facial expression and ability to mimic with Botox, we reduce their capacity to recognize and empathize with feelings.[91]

Empathy is like a muscle that needs to be trained to stay in shape. It is a more passive state, while compassion is linked to the motivation to take action and relieve suffering. Compassion requires empathy but goes a step further with the desire to make the suffering person feel better.

In Buddhist philosophy, our basic nature is called *mind*, and just as water is inherently liquid, our minds have the essential property of being compassionate. Implicit in my discussion of the Self in psychology above was a separation of our experience of "self" and some feeling of an "other," a subject "I" and an object such as another person's body, a table, or aspects of ourselves that we perceive more as objects (i.e., my hand or face). This duality and separation of experiences is a logical way of approaching the world. It helps us navigate the consensus reality and Dreaming aspects of the world. But to tap into our intrinsically compassionate minds, to experience consciousness and the organizing principles behind the world of subjects and objects, to appreciate the music of our bodies, we need to go beyond dualistic thinking and relate to the essence or Process Mind level, a state of creative emptiness or thought-free wakefulness.[92] Many meditation practices and prayers can help us connect to this level. Below, we will practice space-time Dreaming as an alternative way.

Our bodies and brains are central to constructing our worlds and experiences. Our underlying mental processes give rise to bites of information, which our consciousness turns into a coherent narrative like a film that is created on the screen of our videos. Consciousness and Mind are the light and energy that throw the images onto the screen. Our world is inside out: created from the inside with ongoing input and feedback from the outside. What creates the experience of music, a film, New York, "I am," remains a mystery. Nevertheless, it is a mystery that we can experience through meditation, prayer, and space-time Dreaming.

We are not our thoughts and images of who we are. Our true nature is probably more related to the Mind or power that feeds the computer and generates the mental processes. Some say that our experiences are formed and tangible but not real, whereas this Mind principle is formless and not tangible, but real. Many religious, spiritual, mindfulness, and meditation practices are geared toward helping us connect with this Mind principle, which is also called Buddha mind, the Self, God, essence, and more. From that perspective, we are already and always whole and healthy. Accessing our Process Mind connects us with our innate health.

Religions and spiritual traditions have explained the creation and design of the universe in terms of a God or gods. Arnold Mindell coined the term *Process Mind* to describe this wisdom. He based his discussion of Process Mind on his understanding of physics and psychology and by listening to the stories of people who, in nature, in their dreams, their creativity, their altered states and peak experiences, come into contact with some intelligence that is larger than themselves.

There are different ways of connecting to our Process Mind. One is space-time Dreaming, which we will practice later. Empathy, as we have seen, is mediated through a process of mirroring other people's feelings. Reflecting is a third.

Our environment and the people around us reflect back to us who we are. In psychology we call this *projection*; we project aspects of ourselves onto others and learn more about ourselves through the reflection that comes back. Jung called another process of reflection *synchronicity*: events with no causal relationship but some meaningful connection. Synchronistic incidents bring a complementary meaning to a situation and a reflection of Process Mind. Mindell calls these *flirts*: aspects and events in our environment that subconsciously speak to us. Our attention catches them briefly, but we tend to neglect them. These are Dreaming and essence aspects of ourselves. I, for example, have an uncanny ability to spot whales on the Oregon beach, and my wife, Kara, senses turtles before she can see them swimming in the water. Mirroring and reflection happen in all sensory channels: sight, in perceiving and mirroring facial expressions; sound, through sounds that "flirt" with us or that we imitate; touch, through empathic body feelings; and taste and smell, through olfactory experiences that carry meaningful associations.

Our body symptoms, wounds, cracks, and faults are one more process of reflection: They show us another side of ourselves and ultimately can help us connect to our Process Mind. With curiosity, empathy, and compassion, we can include them in our quest to discover who we are and connect to our basic and true nature. Marie Louise Von Franz said that they represent the wounded healer as an archetype of the Self.[93] We naturally connect and equate trauma, wounds, and body symptoms with suffering and damage. But suffering can be the making of somebody, trauma can be transformed into emotional strength, misfortune can lend life quality, and body symptoms can be the root of growth and development. Not all pain is treatable or needs to be treated. Not all body symptoms can be or need to be cured. A treatment and helping-focused mentality can miss the opportunity for bridging the world of consensus reality together with Dreaming and Process Mind.

Presence

Before I delve into space-time Dreaming, the practice to connect with Process Mind, I want to examine more deeply the concept of Presence. I concluded Chapter 9 with Brené Brown's reference to the ministry of Presence, the building of community through the process of sharing pain and processing trauma. The social psychologist Amy Cuddy[94] discusses the power of Presence on an individual level. For her, Presence speaks to one's ability to convey comfort, confidence, and enthusiasm; she believes this ability to be based on feeling connected to one's core values and true self. This Presence is contagious and is correlated with being sought after for jobs and other measures of mainstream success. In her research, she found that this trait is rare and that many people feel less powerful, experience self-criticism, and think they are impostors even while successfully achieving their goals.

But if we ground ourselves in the truth of our own stories, as she recommends, we find that our journeys through life are paved with windy roads and complex, difficult, and sometimes traumatic experiences. Our true selves are fraught with suffering, self-doubts, and insecurities, as well as moments of being attuned to and aligned with a sense of feeling good and at home in ourselves.

Cuddy recommends practicing specific power poses for two minutes as a way to occupy the feeling of being powerful. Mind-body research has shown that body postures affect certain hormones, such as testosterone (an assertiveness hormone) and cortisol (a stress hormone), and that these, in turn, influence how we feel.[95] In other words, the way we feel emotionally translates into physiological states and body expressions, and vice versa. Bringing awareness to our body postures helps us gain consciousness about momentary feelings, which, in turn, allows us to shift our inner experiences by making physical changes.

Body Language and Communication

We conduct whole conversations through our body language, both with others and ourselves. Our body expressions and signals reveal how we feel and who we are. They are often incongruent with how we consciously present ourselves. For example, when two heads of state shake their hands sealing an agreement they just made, while at the same time turning away from each other, you can see the insincerity in their body language.

These double signals (one conscious signal saying one thing, and another less-conscious signal saying something else) are pervasive and universal. They are the expression of conflicting feelings and tendencies. They are predictive of outcomes. They are the manifestation of the whole story, which is often more complicated than what we want to acknowledge.

To ground ourselves in the truth of our whole stories, I recommend bringing forth the conflicting sides—the yesses and the noes, the wants and dislikes, the feelings of "I am able to do this" and "I am not able to do this." Our deepest, most authentic selves and essence often encompass both potentialities. Truth and trust come from being congruent in both verbal and body language. But we are often unaware that we are not representing ourselves fully and truly. Cultural, gender, and other socializing factors push us to think we should be behaving in a certain way or speaking in a particular way.

Amy Cuddy applies her concept of Presence to the consensus reality dimension of our lives, which is very relevant for many of us who struggle to find our places in life and fight the abuse of power and other traumas. However, this is small medicine. In Big Medicine, Presence goes a step further, helping us to ground in the truth and meaning of our whole stories. As von Franz explained, our wounded selves are our true Selves. Healing, in a holistic or Big Medicine sense, comes through the processing of suffering, wounds, and injuries.

Space-Time Dreaming

Space-time Dreaming is a practice of connecting to our Process Minds. It is a method that echoes and has common elements with other spiritual and psychological traditions such as self-remembering (Gurdjieff),[96] radical acceptance (Linehan), the God within (Purusha), Mushin (or creative mind), wu wei, Hineni, presencing (Scharmer), and many other concepts and approaches.

Self-remembering, one of Gurdjieff's main teachings, is at times called *self-consciousness* or *self-presence*. Like Buddhist mindfulness, it is a practice that aims at bridging our experience of the inner and outer world. Outside and inside world are perceived together as a unity of experiences. It is the practice of directly feeling one's aliveness in the present moment—an awareness of being here, now, fully present. One is aware of, for example, the feeling of anger and the "I" who is angry. It is the perception of both the outside and inside world in a unified and embodied way. It is about becoming aware of the auto-pilot in us that does things automatically while also remembering the "I" that is in the driver's seat. We usually identify with our thoughts, feelings, and sensations and are not in contact with the "I" that is doing the thinking, having the feelings, and receiving the perceptions. This self-remembering requires a global attention that is simultaneously aware of body, mind, and feeling.

In Hindu philosophy, Purusha is the universal principle of nature that animates cause and effect. It is the soul of the universe—the universal spirit that is present everywhere, in everything and everyone, at all times. Purusha contrasts with Prakriti, the material reality that constantly changes. In yoga, Purusha is a term meaning "the true self."

In Zen Buddhism, *mushin* is a mind that is not fixed or occupied by thought or emotion and is thus open to everything; it is sometimes called *empty mind* or *creative mind*. It is the mind working with no conscious intention, direction, or plan; a state of openness to the inherent flow. *Wu wei* is a concept in Taoism of being wholly in harmony with the Tao, of following the natural flow without striving—a state of effortless doing, of non-action and following the harmony that already exists.

In the Jewish tradition, Abraham responds to the call of God by stating "Hineni," meaning "here I am." Hineni refers to being present and attentive to God's will.

Presencing blends *presence* and *sensing*. It means stepping into our authentic self and connecting with the Source. It is about coming from the knowing field, relating to the essence, and sensing what wants to come forth.[97]

Radical acceptance is about accepting life on life's terms. It is accepting something from the depth of your soul, in your mind, heart, and body; accepting reality for what it is; and following the rules of the universe.[98]

All these concepts, and no doubt more, describe the same intention and attitude: to be present in the moment, mindful of our actions, and living from a place of understanding and essence. This often requires a change in consciousness—leaving an everyday state and connecting to a source of knowing that is bigger than ourselves: God, Nature, the Self, or Purusha. Process Mind describes this universal organizing principle. To get there, we must relax our mind, detach from the entanglement of opposing forces and tendencies, and let ourselves be moved by the universe.

Exercise: Space-Time Dreaming

The space-time Dreaming practice below is an easy mindfulness exercise that helps you get to that place and find new perspectives:[99]

1. What is your worst health problem?
2. Identify what disturbs you most about this problem. Is it pain, some impairment, lack of energy, fear of death?
3. Explore that experience in more depth. Give it space and discover its energetic quality. Make a hand gesture and energy sketch that captures this quality.[100] Call it X-energy.
4. Now step into the part in you that dislikes the disturbing experience. What is that part of you about—going about life, completing a project, being with your family? Make a hand gesture and energy sketch that captures this quality.[101] Call it u-energy.
5. In your mind, go to your favorite spot on earth, a place you feel most at home. Reconnect with that place and look around and use all your senses to experience what it is like there. See if you can find representations of both the X- and u-energies.
6. Now close your eyes, relax your shoulders, and let your mind become slightly altered. Stand up (if you can) and in your mind rise above the earth spot into the universe. Let space or gravity move you unpredictably and step into its dance by following the repeating moving patterns. Let the dance explain how X- and u-energies are connected in the oneness of the Process Mind.[102]

I will give a personal example. Currently, my worst health problem is a spasm that I experience in my esophagus when I eat certain dry foods too fast and am somehow stressed by the circumstances. It happened to me again just two nights ago. When this spasm happens, nothing goes down my esophagus, not even saliva, and it makes me choke. In the past, I have often had to go to the emergency room to get a muscle relaxant and relieve the spasm. Then a nurse told me a trick with Coca-Cola that has the same effect (see also Chapter 6).

The spasm is most distressing to me, as it makes me choke and doesn't allow me to swallow at all. As I remember the experience, I make a fist that holds my esophagus tightly. The fist has total control over me. In the sketch I draw, I see focus and control. This is my X-energy.

The spasm hinders me from swallowing, from continuing along with eating and everything else I am set up to do. My easygoing side, which prefers to follow along and not disturb the peace, is most upset with my own marginalized X-energy. The sketch of my u-energy depicts a faint wave that moves along.

My favorite spot on earth is Strawberry Hill, a State park on the Oregon coast. The cove beach is secluded and surrounded by forested hills, with some prominent lava rocks that part the waters. The lava rocks remind me of my X-energy, and I see the u-energy in the ripples that the water and sand make. In my space-time dance, I move like a drunk, stumbling with no specific direction. In the stumbling, there are some unpredictable little bursts of energy and stronger movements. In between I sway slowly, altered and inward, sensing more than doing.

The dance shows me a way of being, with unpredictable outbursts of strength spaced by moments of inwardness and introspection. Through my dance, I have now accessed my Process Mind, and it has shown me how these two seemingly disparate energies are meant to relate to one another. This helps me understand basic behavioral patterns that I know I engage in. I am very often more introverted, but I also experience bouts of strength, power, and assertiveness.

An alternate way of relating to the Process Mind expressed in a symptom is by metaphorically following the symptom experience back to its original beginning. Start with the full manifestation of the most disturbing symptom quality (for me, the spasm), and in your mind, go backward to what you imagine was its very beginning. Do so by expressing the energy in a gesture with your hand and then slowly making the gesture smaller and smaller with the aim of capturing the initial intent or impulse of the gesture. My spasm becomes a little and light initiating tap, a small stimulus that gives me direction. You will ask: What does this have to do with the esophagus spasm and medicine? Isn't it easier to treat it, get rid of it if possible, or prevent triggering it? Yes—I do all the above as well. And then, this exercise gives me a new way of relating to it, of putting it into a larger context. It's not a foreign body or experience anymore. It becomes more part of me, part of my true self.

It is hard to describe the experience of doing the space-time Dreaming exercise and getting in touch with the Process Mind. These are subtle embodied experiences, forms of pre-sensing and presence. The important part is to allow yourself to go into the altered state of being moved without intention. You get into a meditative movement experience, from where you can catch the unintentional movement flirts and associations that come with them. It's a form of active imagination and accessing unconscious creative spaces. It will make sense to you in a way that is hard to express in words. Try the exercise; it can help you ground yourself in the truth of your own stories and essence.

Chapter 11

CONCLUSION:
BURNOUT AND VICARIOUS RESILIENCE

I N THIS FINAL chapter, I will attempt to join the many strands of Big Medicine, showing how together we can weave a new colorful fabric of health, medicine, and healing.

The main proposition of Big Medicine is that both health and sickness are processes on a journey through life; they are stations on an evolutionary, cyclical path full of wonders and challenges. Throughout the book, we have discussed the pitfalls of a normative approach to health I call "bell curve medicine." We have explored Process, the depth of inner experiences, power and relationship dynamics, and Process Mind. We discovered that Big Medicine is science, art, and a path for spiritual growth. Mind and body are instruments of trauma, suffering, and harm, as well as creativity and intelligence. Our embodied mind and consciousness, with all their strengths and failings, are the manifestation of the Dreammaker, Mushin, the Buddha, Process Mind, or whatever you want to call the mind of God.

The Flu, a Troll, and the Power of Being Present in Your Body

In a recent workshop, I worked with George, who was recovering from a recent flu bug. The virus, he felt, had drained his life force, and he was worried about not getting better. He also mentioned that, paradoxically, he had enjoyed being forced to follow his body's energy and stay in bed. I asked him what, currently, was his most distressing symptom.

He responded that he felt weak. I led him to explore his sense of weakness and follow how his body wanted to move. He immediately slumped in his chair, dropping his shoulders and arms. I encouraged him to believe in the intelligence of his body and follow its natural leaning. He ended on the floor almost lifeless.

I crouched alongside him and assisted him in going deeper into his experience by pacing his breath and engaging in minimal hands-on bodywork. At one point he opened his eyes, looked at me, and got a fright. I asked him what had just happened, and he said he saw me at his side and that I had the expression of a troll. I followed that fantasy, enacting the troll, and I asked him to engage with that scary monster. A lively, playful, and energetic scuffle ensued as we took turns being the troll.

Afterwards, George reflected on how he had relished the physicality and playfulness of the encounter. We pondered how the flu had helped him to be more present in his body and listen to its messages. He ended by exclaiming: "Having the flu, I recommend it!"

Below is a picture of the specific troll George had in mind when he saw me squatting beside him. It is a huge public sculpture underneath the Fremont Bridge in Seattle. It explains the fear it generated in him. George's imaginary troll, the embodiment of the life force he was missing, was there to awaken him to being attuned to his body. The troll reminded me also of the Mucinex TV add that depicts a troll-like figure symbolizing mucus and phlegm. Our Big Medicine exploration of my client's flu symptoms had tapped into a form of active imagination, which in turn sparked archetypical images. God's mind triggered a fantasy of a vicious troll—or it took the face of this creature to reconnect my client with the physicality of his body.

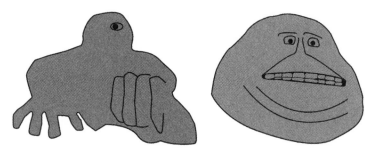

Figure 8. Troll Under the Fremont Bridge in Seattle[103] and Mucinex Troll[104]

Viral infections such as the flu gain a foothold when our immune system breaks down due to stress overload. The now-ubiquitous notion of stress originated in engineering: Building materials were tested for their resistance to outside forces to determine the material's breaking points. Like other materials, the body has its own limits, and when it is exposed to too much emotional and physical strain, its ability to resist the onslaught of challenges fails.

After each year in medical school, I had to complete difficult exams that required hours of memorizing theories and facts. The failure rate of these exams was often higher than 50 percent. Every single year, I was able to sustain the stress of studying, and unfailingly, I fell sick right after the last exam was over. We can push ourselves and our bodies to a certain point and then they revolt and demand to be cared for. The body's reserves have a certain life span before they burn out. Many physical, emotional, and spiritual factors play an important role in regulating our ability to withstand dire circumstances. The 12 teenage Thai soccer players and their coach who were trapped in a pitch-dark flooded cave for nine days without food survived by meditating and by drawing strength from their team spirit. This is a prime example of how our minds can mitigate health challenges.

Aaron Antonovsky, the Israeli sociologist I mentioned in Chapter 4, called our health-promoting faculty *a sense of coherence*. He defined *coherence* as our ability to retain the notion that our present circumstances, no matter how grim, can be managed and that they will turn out to be somehow meaningful. In his research, problems arose when individuals started questioning their faculties to overcome challenges and make them valuable. At this point, they lost hope.

Empathy, Compassion, and Burnout

Burnout is a situation of losing hope. Common among clinicians, it is the feeling of exhaustion and loss of interest that is related to chronic work-related stress, such as feeling overwhelmed with the needs of patients and unable to adequately help. The symptoms of burnout closely match the symptoms of depression. They are a response to outer and inner demands and the expectations that exhaust our mental and physical resources.

Compassion fatigue is a form of burnout in professionals and lay individuals who care more specifically for survivors of trauma, abuse, and illness. It is sometimes called *secondary traumatic stress* or *vicarious trauma*. The symptoms again overlap with those of burnout and depression. These syndromes imply that we have limited resources for giving and caring, that our minds and bodies work like batteries with a finite number of times we can recharge them. Therefore, we need to use our energies wisely and spend time recharging them when they run down to avoid a situation when our batteries eventually lose the ability to hold a charge.

New research shows that compassion and empathy are processed by very different cerebral networks. Empathic reactions activate and correlate with areas of the brain that are associated with pain.[105] We suffer when we see someone suffering. But when focusing on compassion, the brain's networks linked to distress and negative emotions are not activated. Instead, cerebral areas associated with feelings of affiliation and maternal love are. Our empathic resonance with someone else's pain and the compassion we experience for that suffering are emotionally and biologically different.[106] Empathy alerts us that the other is suffering and compassion motivates us to take action. It is the first step that gives us the urge to engage in compassionate love and actively confront other's suffering by better caring for them. Because empathy, or affective resonance with suffering, can be distressing and paralyzing, it can lead to the emotional exhaustion characteristic of burnout. So, the reality is that empathy gets fatigued—not compassion.

Compassion, in contrast, is a positive state that we can train ourselves in. Stanford University, for example, offers a course in compassion cultivation that includes traditional contemplative practices alongside contemporary research on compassion.[107] As I have discussed, not being able to relieve suffering can become its own cause of suffering for providers and caregivers. That is why compassion training also includes training to strengthen compassion toward yourself, reducing stress, improving self-care, and combating unrealistic expectations and negative self-criticism.

When we engage in active compassionate care of someone who is suffering, we often experience that we are gaining something. This contrasts with the experience of empathic distress and burnout. This positive reward is often called *resilience, post-traumatic growth,* or *vicarious resilience.*

Resilience describes someone's ability to stay well despite challenging events and life circumstances. It is the faculty to adapt to adversity and spring back into a prior state of wellness. Resilience is what people who face trauma and stress commonly demonstrate; it is almost normal. Many studies show that community and individual support within and outside of family are what foster resilience. Loving and trusting relationships provide the emotional support needed when facing hardship.

Post-traumatic growth refers to a personal process of change after a traumatic experience that is deeply meaningful. The process includes finding benefits within challenges. When we are witness to another's trauma and suffering, our response can be one of vicarious trauma—feeling overwhelmed and despondent and having intrusive memories and nightmares. Or we can experience a positive response, *vicarious resilience*—feeling inspired and motivated by witnessing the victim's ability to overcome adversity and turn it into a meaningful life story. Victims and their helpers co-create a story that affects them individually and that ripples into their environment and communities.

How Do We Make Sense of a World Full of Trauma?

Efforts to understand the meaning of human suffering are ancient and are central to many religious and spiritual teachings. Suffering and trauma wake us up from slumber and a comfortable life. They give us an advantage in understanding diversity and relating to the human condition. They can also lead to bitterness and resentment.

Big Medicine sees all of it—burnout, compassion fatigue, resilience, growth, bitterness, and resentment—as resting points in a cyclical process of change. They are all meaningful and worthy of awareness and exploration. They are not goals or ends in themselves. They all need our understanding and attention. Burnout and depression may be a call for downtime and introspection; bitterness and resentment may be a first step toward using anger as a motivation to fight more effectively; and resilience may be a momentary ability to be more detached and rise above the distress and suffering.

For Big Medicine, healing and small health are not the only goals. Big Medicine understands that small health is only temporary and restricted to those who have that specific privilege. So, what does a form of medicine look like that is not primarily focused on health and well-being?

From a Big Medicine perspective, an individual health crisis—or, in a larger sense, any illness experience—is a Process Mind emergency. Like vicarious resilience and post-traumatic growth, emotional and physical health challenges offer a path to strengthening coherence and meaning. They are part of our holistic journey through life, and in addition to causing harm, are opportunities for spiritual growth.

Public health disparities and community diversity tensions present a means for the community to develop communal intelligence. Big Medicine is positive medicine and gives us ways to make individual and community life more meaningful and resilient. Big Medicine acknowledges the harm and damage done by disease and community challenges and supports whatever it takes to improve and restore individual, community, and environmental health. Part of this effort includes integrating experiences of illness and community strife. These are not only problems that cause harm—they are also expressions of our individual and community diversity and can ultimately help us strengthen resilience, coherence, and meaning.

Exercise: Burnout as a Form of Resilience

The following exercise is a Big Medicine way of reflecting on burnout and turning it into a process for individual coping and resilience.

1. Sit back, relax, and notice how it feels to be you right now.
2. If you are feeling burned out, tired, depressed,[108] or hopeless, explore the experience with curiosity. If you don't feel burned out right now, remember a time when you felt overwhelmed, fatigued, distressed, or numbed out.
3. Take a moment to study your response to the burnout sensation. Do you need more vacation, time off, or time for yourself? Are there specific issues (individual, relational, social, cultural) that weigh on you that you need to tackle? Make a mental note to plan how you can address whatever you identified.[109]
4. How does the burnout experience feel emotionally, mentally, and in your body? Is it lethargy, "brain freeze," heaviness, emptiness,

anxiety panic, or something else? Uncover that experience with an open mind.

5. Breathe into it and let it engulf you. Give it space and let it move you at its own pace and timing. Embrace the burnout experience.

6. While staying in that experience, let it speak to you through images, feelings, thoughts, and insights.

7. Next, ask yourself who in you needs this burnout medicine. Who needs burnout? What part of you is the experience of burnout meant for?

8. Decide to use the "burnout" experience as your tool for resilience.[110]

I just had a big week of work and experienced another event of dysphagia, or not being able to swallow. Medical support helped me through the distressing incident, and I decided to review some of my dietary habits. This week's U.S. and world political news put another layer of strain on me. The result of all this is a sense of discouragement and drain. I am reminded by my symptom to re-center myself. Following the burnout experience, my body feels heavier and tends to lean backwards. As I go along, I end up lying down and closing my eyes. I feel the gravity and imagine floating on a mattress in the middle of a lake with the sun warming my whole body. The sun tells me to relax and let itself shine through me.

I began, in the Preface to this book, with a powerful statement that posits medicine in a cultural and political context and places my own views and opinions within a frame of reference that is influenced by my social identities and privileges. In this book I have also swayed between looking at individual processes and their cultural embedding and discussing community health matters. The individual and collective intersect; they are powerfully entangled in our bodies' stories.

Big Medicine's use of Dreaming is meant to work with these multidimensional forces. They create a unique, time-bound process that is both individual and collective. Aspects of this process express themselves in our struggles and pleasures with our bodies and their ailments.

This embodied process, in turn, has information that is meaningful for us as individuals and can help us build better communities. Process is, by definition, ever-changing and inclusive of diversity. The body's hidden meanings expand our knowledge of ourselves. It is as if the artist Dreammaker in her secret studio paints us to become more whole and inclusive.

As I was handling my own body's defiance and struggles with allowing me to swallow, I dreamed that I had parked my car in the parking garage of a ski resort. After spending the day enjoying skiing, I was ready to retrieve my car. The parking attendant gave me a ticket with my car's place number, but my car was not in that place. I went back to the attendant and asked him to find my car. Instead, he told me that if I insisted on finding my car, it would cost me a lot of money. Confused and angry, I retorted that I had a lawyer representing me and would happily sue them.

Skiing is one of my favorite activities. I relish the freedom of movement and the snowy expansions I negotiate with my skis as I follow nature's markings. The car is what brings me to this pleasure. I immediately associated it with my body and interpreted the paradoxical message of the attendant as warning me to let go of my old ways of operating. Stubbornly and righteously, I fight back and threaten to sue.

This clash parallels the fight between me wanting to swallow food and the esophageal spasm that stops me. For me, to pursue "skiing," I need a new mode of transport and operating. I also find myself in a struggle with my doctors, who want me to take strong antacid and anti-inflammatory medicine. In some ways, this is a reasonable medical approach, one that I am trained in. But the proposed medications have some significant long-term side effects, many of which interfere with digestion. What a beautiful and impossible mess. To go against medical advice, I found out, is psychologically complicated for me. It goes against my training and identity. Here again, I find myself confronted with contradiction and differing ideas.

When I enter the mindset of the Dreammaker who produces the

spasm, I am reminded to become more conscious of what I swallow and of how and what I eat. It forces me to step out of my unconscious habits and to change my modus operandi. In my night dream, I don't get a new car or find a new way. I do hear the warning that it will cost me a lot if I heed the old ways. It's an evolving process.

With Big Medicine I aspire to follow my calling and passion about medicine and Process. It personifies the belief for a necessary change in matters of health, healthcare, medicine, our views of bodies, and their different conditions. As it touches on matters of life and death, pain, trauma, community, and environment, Big Medicine is a spiritual quest and adventure. Medicine and health are about Process. Diseases and ill health are problems that need our attention. And they are also gifts that remind us of our deeper selves.

I close with the thoughts of my client Julia, who came to me for help processing her experiences around advanced smooth muscle cancer. With extreme courage and tenacity, she approached her cancer as an opportunity for inner transformation. Julia passed away in February 2019.

> *Healing is a poem written with the language of symptoms.*
> *Its rhythm is energy, is life, is what cannot yet be understood.*
> *The body calls for a different language: You have to enter*
> *the unknown. This is a sign of the intelligence of the soul.*

NOTES

1) For example, Western medicine's widespread use of hormones and antibiotics have significant effects on livestock and the environment.

2) Our inner world reflects the diversity of the world outside. As we internalize the norms and values of our communities, we tend to embrace dominant beliefs and reject others. The marginalized parts of ourselves might then show up in body symptoms or other unintentional or secondary processes. For instance, a chronic headache might reflect a suppressed assertiveness, while an autoimmune disorder could mirror internal and external gender-based oppression.

3) *Nature* with a capital "N" refers to Mother Nature as the organizing principle or the source and guiding force of creation.

4) Pierre Morin, *Health in Sickness, Sickness in Health* (Portland: Deep Democracy Exchange, 2014).

5) For further exploration of the intersection between the community and the body, see Chapter 8.

6) Aaron Antonovsky, *Health, Stress, and Coping: New Perspectives on Mental and Physical Well-Being* (San Francisco: Jossey-Bass, 1979), 122.

7) For more information, check out our Facebook page at https://www.facebook.com/dreambodymedicine/.

8) Ivan Illich, "Health as One's Own Responsibility—No, Thank You!"

based on a speech given in Hanover, Germany, September 14, 1990, trans. Jutta Mason, ed. Lee Hoinacki, https://www.scribd.com/document/2910760/1990-health-responsibility-Ivan-Illich, accessed July 29, 2018.

9) World Health Organization, *Adherence to long-term therapies: evidence for action* (Geneva: World Health Organization, 2003), http://www.who.int/chp/knowledge/publications/adherence_full_report.pdf, accessed October 5, 2018.

10) The concept of *mainstreaming* comes from the U.S. educational system, where it refers to placing children with disabilities in regular classrooms. I use it to describe the process of adjusting to and adopting mainstream values and notions of beauty, fitness, and health; the process of looking in the mirror and making corrections to your appearance, or of standing on a scale and resolving to start a diet. It is one of the main sources for self-hatred.

11) Andrew Solomon, *Far from the Tree* (New York: Scribner, 2012).

12) Meghan O'Rourke, "What's Wrong with Me? I had an autoimmune disease. Then the disease had me," *The New Yorker,* August 26, 2013, https://www.newyorker.com/magazine/2013/08/26/whats-wrong-with-me, accessed September 27, 2018.

13) Avraham Cohen, "Becoming a Daoist Educator," in *Speaking of Teaching,* eds. Avraham Cohen, Marion Porath, and Anthony Clarke (Rotterdam: Sense Publishers, 2013): 26–27.

14) Friedrich Wilhelm Nietzsche, *The Gay Science* (Minneola: Dover Publications, 2006).

15) Personal comments made by Arnold Mindell during his Friday class, September 9, 2017 in Portland, Oregon.

16) For a more in-depth exploration of this topic, see the book I co-wrote with my friend Gary Reiss, *Inside Coma: A New View of Awareness, Healing and Hope* (Santa Barbara: Praeger, 2010).

17) Vincent J. Felitti et al., "Relationship of Childhood Abuse and Household Dysfunction to Many of the Leading Causes of Death

in Adults. The Adverse Childhood Experiences (ACE) Study," *American Journal of Preventive Medicine*, 14(1998): 245–258.

18) Arnold Mindell, *Process Mind: A User's Guide to Connecting to the Mind of God* (Wheaton: Quest Books, 2010).

19) Thomas Mann, *The Coming Victory of Democracy* (New York: Alfred A. Knopf, Inc., 1938).

20) Naturopathic and alternative treatment modalities such as herbs, homeopathy, acupuncture, chiropractic, Reiki, etc. have different ways of conceptualizing health and sickness. Many adhere to some form of differentiation between a state of balance and health and a state of imbalance and sickness. When used as treatments toward achieving a state of wellness and health, they pertain to the consensus reality level.

21) Arnold Mindell, *The Dreammaker's Apprentice: Using Heightened States of Consciousness to Interpret Dreams* (Charlottesville: Hampton Roads Publishing Company Inc., 2001).

22) Arnold Mindell, *Process Mind: A User's Guide to Connecting with the Mind of God* (Wheaton: Quest Books, 2010): 42.

23) Aaron Antonovsky, *Health, Stress and Coping: New Perspectives on Mental and Physical Well-Being* (San Francisco: Jossey-Bass Publishers, 1979).

24) Viktor Frankl, *Man's Search for Meaning. An Introduction to Logotherapy* (Boston: Beacon Press, 2006).

25) George E. Vaillant referenced in Carolyn Gregoire, "The 75-Year Study That Found the Secrets to a Fulfilling Life," *The Huffington Post*, August 23, 2013, https://www.huffingtonpost.com/2013/08/11/how-this-harvard-psycholo_n_3727229.html, accessed April 24, 2018.

26) George E. Vaillant, *Triumphs of Experience: The Men of the Harvard Grant Study* (Cambridge: Belknap Press, 2012).

27) Jacob Needleman, "Questions of the Heart. Inner Empiricism as a Way to a Science of Consciousness," *Noetic Sciences Review* (Summer

1993), http://cogweb.ucla.edu/Abstracts/Needleman _93.html, accessed September 27, 2018.

28) Thomas Merton quoted in J. Conner, "The Original Face in Buddhism and the True Self of Thomas Merton," *Cistercian Studies*, 22(4) (1987): 343–351.

29) D. Harrison, "Complementarity and the Copenhagen Interpretation of Quantum Mechanics," *Upscale*, March 27, 2006, https://faraday. physics.utoronto.ca/GeneralInterest/Harrison/Complementarity/ CompCopen.html, accessed September 27, 2018.

30) Michael Pollan, *Cooked: A Natural History of Transformation* (New York: Penguin Books, 2013).

31) Blaise Pascal (1623–1662), "On Busyness, Distraction and Diversion," https://deovivendiperchristum.wordpress.com/2013/ 07/30/ blaise-pascal-1623-1662-on-busyness-distraction-and-diversion/, accessed September 27, 2018.

32) Aaron Antonovsky, *Health, Stress and Coping: New Perspectives on Mental and Physical Well-Being* (San Francisco: Jossey-Bass, 1979).

33) Eugene Gendlin, *Focusing* (New York: Bantam [revised edition] 1981): 10.

34) F.J. Varela, E. Thompson, and E. Rosch, *The Embodied Mind: Cognitive Science and Human Experience* (Cambridge: MIT Press, 1991).

35) Jalal al-Din Rumi, *The Essential Rumi*, trans. Coleman Barks (San Francisco: Harper, 2004).

36) Amy Mindell, *Metaskills: The Spiritual Art of Therapy* (Tempe: New Falcon 1994/2001).

37) "Lost Mothers. Nothing Protects Black Women from Dying in Pregnancy and Childbirth," *ProPublica*, https://www.propublica. org/ article/nothing-protects-black-women-from-dying-in-pregnancy-and-childbirth, accessed September 27, 2018.

38) Michelle Alexander, "Who We Want to Become: Beyond the New Jim Crow," https://www.onbeing.org/program/michelle-alexander-who-we-want-to-become-beyond-the-new-jim-crow/transcript/ 8611, accessed September 27, 2018.

39) *The Divide: What Happens When the Rich Get Richer?* https:// thedivideddocumentary.com/, accessed September 27, 2018.

40) Martin Daly, *Killing the Competition: Economic Inequality and Homicide* (New Brunswick: Transaction Publishers, 2016).

41) "US County Profile: Baltimore County," (Maryland: Institute for Health Metrics and Evaluation, 2016).

42) Karl Marx, *The 18th Brumaire of Louis Bonaparte* (Cabin John: Wildside Press, 2008).

43) M.G. Marmot et al. "Health Inequalities Among British Civil Servants: the Whitehall II Study," *Lancet* 337(8754) (1991): 1387–1393.

44) Amartya Sen, *Development as Freedom* (New York: Alfred A. Knopf Inc., 1999).

45) The Princeton economists Anne Case and Angus Deaton found that the death rate of middle-aged white American men without a college degree has increased since the 1990s. This is in contrast to the increase in life expectancy of the average population. This generation of poor white men is experiencing widening income inequality and stagnant social mobility. Prior generations could count on more opportunities, some upward mobility, and more affluence. The unfulfilled expectations and the experience of performing poorly in comparison to their parents and others around them contributes to this group of white men making unhealthy choices and dying from cirrhosis of the liver, suicide, and overdose of opiates and painkillers. Anne Case and Angus Deaton, "Rising Morbidity and Mortality in Midlife Among White non-Hispanic Americans in the 21st Century," *Proceedings of the National Academy of Sciences (PNAS)* 112(49) (December 2015): 15078–15083.

46) J.E. Ferrie, "Work, Stress and Health: Findings from the Whitehall II Study," *Occupational Health Review* 111(2004): 20–21.

47) N. Snyder-Mackler et al., "Social Status Alters Immune Regulation and Response to Infection in Macaques," *Science* 354(6315) (November 2016): 1041–1045.

48) S.E. Taylor, "Tend and Befriend: Biobehavioral Bases of Affiliation

Under Stress," *Current Directions in Psychological Science* 15(6) (2006).

49) M.J. Meaney, "Maternal Care, Gene Expression, and the Transmission of Individual Difference in Stress Reactivity Across Generations," *Annual Review of Neuroscience* 24 (2001): 1161–92.

50) B. Lask, C. Britten C, L. Kroll, J. Magagna J, and M. Tranter, "Children with Pervasive Refusal," *Archives of Disease in Childhood* 66 (1991): 866–869.

51) Rachel Aviv, "The Trauma of Facing Deportation," *The New Yorker*, April 3, 2017, https://www.newyorker.com/magazine/ 2017/04/ 03/the-trauma-of-facing-deportation, accessed August 31, 2018.

52) For a more in-depth discussion of rank, see Chapter 9.

53) Daniel Goleman, *Emotional Intelligence* (New York: Bantam Books Inc. 1995).

54) Howard Gardner proposed the theory of multiple intelligences. He defines *intelligence* as the "biopsychological potential to process information that can be activated in a cultural setting to solve problems or create products that are of value in a culture." According to Gardner, we can do this through more than just logical and linguistic intelligence. He explores interpersonal intelligence, social intelligence (the capability to effectively navigate complex social relationships), and moral, spiritual, and existential intelligences. Howard Gardner, *Intelligence Reframed: Multiple Intelligences for the 21st Century* (New York: Basic Books, 1999): 33–34.

Another term used in the fields of political science and sociobiology is *collective intelligence,* also written as *collective IQ.* Collective intelligence can be understood as the shared group intelligence that comes from collaborating and building consensus. It is an emergent property that arises from the combined forces and intelligences of individual group or community members. It shifts the power and knowledge from the individual to the collective.

The idea that multiple intelligences are required to navigate life's challenges and find value and meaning is also relevant in our discussion of health and medicine. Communal intelligence is an individual trait, whereas collective intelligence is a trait that arises within a group.

55) See also the section on communing in Chapter 5.

56) The concept of communal intelligence is defined as an individual trait. A group of highly communally intelligent people can have a great impact on community dialogues.

57) Ivan Van Sertima (ed.), *Golden Age of the Moors* (Livingston: Transaction Publishers, 1992).

58) Damon Tweedy, "The Case for Black Doctors," *The New York Times*, May 15, 2015, https://www.nytimes.com/2015/05/17/opinion/sunday/ the-case-for-black-doctors.html, accessed August 26, 2018.

59) Ibid.

60) Chokyi Nyima Rinpoche with David R. Shlim, MD, *Medicine & Compassion: A Tibetan Lama's Guidance for Caregivers* (Somerville: Winston Publications, 2006).

61) For an in-depth review of the neuroscience of relationships, see: Daniel J. Siegel, *The Developing Mind. How Relationships and the Brain Interact to Shape Who We Are, 2nd ed* (New York: The Guilford Press, 2012).

62) C.N. DeWall et al., "Acetaminophen Reduces Social Pain: Behavioral and Neural Evidence," *Psychological Science* 21(7) (2010): 931–937.

63) John Kabat-Zinn, *Mindfulness Meditation for Pain Relief: Guided Practices for Reclaiming Your Body and Your Life* Audiobook, https://www.audible.com.

64) For a review of the science of presence, see: S. Parker, B. Nelson, E. Epel, and D. Siegel, "The Science of Presence: A Central Mediator of the Interpersonal Benefits of Mindfulness," in *Handbook of Mindfulness: Theory, Research, and Practice*, ed. K.W. Brown, J.D. Creswell, R.M. Ryan (New York: The Guilford Press, 2015).

65) Shari M. Geller, *A Practical Guide to Cultivating Therapeutic Presence* (Washington: American Psychological Association, 2017).

66) See also Chapter 10.

67) Daniel J. Siegel, *Clinical Applications of Interpersonal Neurobiology* (Psychotherapy Networker, 2013), https://www.psychotherapynetworker. org/ store/detail/14950/the-clinical-applications-of-interpersonal-neurobiology, accessed September 15, 2018.

68) Vilayanur S. Ramachandran, *The Neurology of Self-Awareness* (The Edge, 2007), http://edge.org/conversation/the-neurology-of-self-awareness, accessed September 15, 2018.

69) See also Chapter 8.

70) Social anthropologist Pierre Bourdieu coined the term *habitus* to describe a person's socially familiar ways of perceiving, interpreting, and responding to social cues. Pierre Bourdieu, *Outline of a Theory of Practice* (New York: Cambridge University Press, 1977).

71) Atul Gawande, "Curiosity and What Equality Really Means," *The New Yorker,* https://www.newyorker.com/news/news-desk/curiosity-and-the-prisoner/, accessed June 17, 2018.

72) G. Vaillant and K. Mukamal, "Successful Aging," *American Journal of Psychiatry* 158(2001): 839–847; Vincent J. Felitti et. al., "Relationship of Childhood Abuse and Household Dysfunction to Many of the Leading Causes of Death in Adults: The Adverse Childhood Experiences (ACE) Study," *American Journal of Preventive Medicine* 14(4) (1998): 245–258; M. G. Marmot et al., "Health Inequalities among British civil servants: the Whitehall II study," *Lancet* 337(8754) (1991): 1387–1393.

73) R.M. Puhl and C.A. Heuer, "Obesity Stigma: Important Considerations for Public Health," *Am J Public Health* 100(6) (2010): 1019–1028.

74) A.R. Sutin, Y. Stephan, and A. Terracciano, "Weight Discrimination and Risk of Mortality," *Psychological Science,* 26(11) (2015): 1803-1811.

75) Robin DiAngelo, "White Fragility," *International Journal of Critical Pedagogy*, 3(3) (2011): 54-70.

76) D. Kahan, "Ideology, Motivated Reasoning, and Cognitive Reflection," *Judgment & Decision Making* 407(2013).

77) Brené Brown, *Braving the Wilderness: The Quest for True Belonging and the Courage to Stand Alone* (New York: Random House, 2017).

78) Michele Gelfand, Joshua Conrad Jackson, and Jesse R. Harrington, "Trump Culture: Threat, Fear and the Tightening of the American Mind," *Scientific American*, April 27, 2016, https://www.scientificamerican.com/article/trump-culture-threat-fear-and-the-tightening-of-the-american-mind/, accessed November 29, 2018.

79) Karen Stenner, *The Authoritarian Dynamic* (Cambridge: Cambridge University Press, 2005).

80) Atul Gawande, "Curiosity and What Equality Really Means," *The New Yorker*, June 2, 2018, https://www.newyorker.com/news/news-desk/ curiosity-and-the-prisoner, accessed June 17, 2018.

81) Ijeoma Oluo, *So You Want to Talk About Race* (New York: Seal Press, 2018).

82) Robin DiAngelo, *White Fragility: Why It's So Hard for White People to Talk About Racism* (Boston: Beacon Press, 2018), 20.

83) "Scientists Start to Tease Out The Subtler Ways Racism Hurts Health," https://www.npr.org/sections/health-shots/2017/11/11/562623815/scientists-start-to-tease-out-the-subtler-ways-racism-hurts-health, accessed November 29, 2018.

84) Brené Brown, *Braving the Wilderness: The Quest for True Belonging and the Courage to Stand Alone* (New York: Random House, 2017).

85) John O'Donohue, "Before the Dawn I Begot You: Reflections on Priestly Identity," *The Furrow*, 57(9) (September 2006): 471.

86) Pierre Morin, *Health in Sickness, Sickness in Health* (Portland: Deep Democracy Exchange, 2014).

87) Anil Seth, "How Your Brain Hallucinates Your Conscious Reality,"

TED Talk, 2017. https://www.ted.com/talks/anil_seth_how_your_ brain_hallucinates_your_conscious_reality, accessed September 15, 2018.

88) An example of how the brain predicts information is the "checkershadow illusion." This is an optical illusion documented in 1995 by Edward H. Adelson, professor of vision science at MIT. The image depicts a checkerboard with light and dark squares, partly shadowed by another object. The optical illusion is that the area labeled A appears to be a darker color than the area labeled B. However, within the context of the two-dimensional image, they are of identical shade. "Checkershadow Illusion," http://persci. mit.edu/ gallery/checkershadow, accessed September 15, 2018.

89) The rubber hand illusion is an example of this. In this experiment, human participants view a dummy hand being stroked with a paintbrush while they feel a series of identical brushstrokes applied to their own hand, which is hidden from view. If this visual and tactile information is applied synchronously, and if the visual appearance and position of the dummy hand is similar to the participant's own hand, then the participant feels that the touches on their own hand are coming from the dummy hand, and even that the dummy hand is, in some way, their own hand. M. Botvinick and J. Cohen, "Rubber Hands 'Feel' Touch That Eyes See," *Nature* 391 (1998): 756.

90) T. Kruger and A. Wollmer, "Can Botulinum Toxin Alleviate Symptoms of Borderline Personality Disorder?" Abstract presented at the *American Psychiatric Association Annual Meeting* (New York: May 7, 2018), https://www.psychcongress.com/article/botox-reduces-treatment-resistant-symptoms-bpd, accessed September 15, 2018.

91) D.T. Neal and T.L. Chartrand, "Embodied Emotion Perception: Amplifying and Dampening Facial Feedback Modulates Emotion Perception Accuracy," *Social Psychological and Personality Science* 2(6) (2011): 673–678.

92) From a Buddhist perspective, in the space of openness, where we can

let go of duality and any concepts, true non-conceptual compassion becomes manifest. This form of compassion is spontaneous, natural, and effortless. It is impartial and doesn't distinguish between friend or enemy. In a relaxed state of mind, we are less limited by our own thoughts and emotions. Our true nature has the basic property of compassion. For an in-depth review of compassion and medicine, see Chokyi Nyima Rinpoche and David R. Shlim, *Medicine & Compassion* (Somerville: Wisdom Publications, 2006).

93) Marie-Louise von Franz, "The Process of Individuation," in *Man and His Symbols,* ed. Carl G. Jung (New York: Doubleday Publ., 1964).

94) Amy Cuddy, *Presence: Bringing Your Boldest Self to Your Biggest Challenges* (New York: Back Bay Books, 2015).

95) D.R. Carney, A.J. Cuddy, and A.J. Yap, "Power Posing: Brief Non-verbal Displays Affect Neuroendocrine Levels and Risk Tolerance," *Psychological Science* 21(10) (2010): 1–6.

96) Robert Earl Burton, *Self-Remembering* (York Beach: Samuel Weiser Inc., 1995).

97) "Presencing," Scharmer, http://www.ottoscharmer.com/sites/default/files/TU2_Chapter11.pdf, accessed April 25, 2018.

98) "Radical Acceptance Part 1," Linehan, http://www.dbtselfhelp.com/html/radical_acceptance_part_1.html, accessed April 25, 2018.

99) I recommend reading the exercise along with my personal example below before trying it yourself.

100) For example, pain might have an energy of stabbing or cutting, whereas death might have an energy of going downward, relaxing, or dissolving. Impaired breathing might feel like a constraining pressure.

101) For example, the experience of going about one's life might have a feeling quality of a rhythmical pacing.

102) The movements that you express in your space-time dance have different patterns and qualities. Some will mirror your X- and u-energies. The way your specific dance brings these different patterns together relates to your Process Mind.

103) "Fremont Troll," Wikipedia, https://en.wikipedia.org/wiki/ Fremont_Troll, accessed December 17, 2018.

104) "Images of Mucinex Character," https://www.bing.com/images/ search?q=mucinex+character&qpvt=mucinex+character&FORM =IGRE, accessed December 17, 2018.

105) For a summary of the 32 studies on empathy with regard to pain, see C. Lamm, J. Decety, and T. Singer, "Meta-Analytic Evidence for Common and Distinct Neural Networks Associated with Directly Experienced Pain and Empathy for Pain," *Neuroimage*, 54(3) (2011): 2492–2502.

106) For a neural distinction between compassion and empathy fatigue, see O. Klimecki and T. Singer, "Empathic Distress Fatigue Rather Than Compassion Fatigue? Integrating findings from empathy research in psychology and social neuroscience." In *Pathological Altruism*, edited by B. Oakley, A. Knafo, G. Madhavan, and D.S. Wilson (Oxford University Press, 2011): 368–383.

107) See "About Compassion Cultivation Training," http://ccare.stanford. edu/education/about-compassion-cultivation-training-cct/, and for a scientific review of compassion cultivation, see "Peer-Reviewed Care Articles," http://ccare.stanford.edu/research/ peer-reviewed-ccare-articles/.

108) If you feel strongly depressed and have thoughts of harming yourself, please contact your primary care provider or counselor; if you can't reach them, please go to the nearest emergency room or urgent care clinic.

109) After you have completed this exercise, come back to this step and plan how you can address what you identified as a current need to care for yourself and address your burnout.

110) The insight you get from embracing the burnout state is a powerful tool you can integrate into your everyday life. The image I received, of floating on a lake, helps me relax and let go whenever I remember it. I keep a related picture on top of my work desk.

BIBLIOGRAPHY

Abbass, Allan, and Howard Schubiner. *Hidden from View: A Clinician's Guide to Psychophysiologic Disorders.* Psychophysiologic Press, LLC, 2018.

Antonovsky, Aaron. *Health, Stress and Coping: New Perspectives on Mental and Physical Well-Being.* San Francisco: Jossey-Bass, 1979.

———. *Unraveling the Mystery of Health: How People Manage Stress and Stay Well.* San Francisco: Jossey-Bass, 1987.

Bedrick, David. *Talking Back to Dr. Phil: Alternatives to Mainstream Psychology.* Santa Fe: Belly Song Press, 2013.

———. *Revisioning Activism: Bringing Depth, Dialogue, and Diversity to Individual and Social Change.* Santa Fe: Belly Song Press, 2017.

Bourdieu, Pierre. *Outline of a Theory of Practice.* New York: Cambridge University Press, 1977.

Brown, Brené. *Braving the Wilderness: The Quest for True Belonging and the Courage to Stand Alone.* New York: Random House, 2017.

Burton, Robert Earl. *Self-Remembering.* York Beach: Samuel Weiser Inc., 1995.

Cuddy, Amy. *Presence: Bringing Your Boldest Self to Your Biggest Challenges.* New York: Back Bay Books, 2015.

Daly, Martin. *Killing the Competition: Economic Inequality and Homicide.* New Brunswick: Transaction Publishers, 2016.

Davanloo, Habib. *Intensive Short-Term Dynamic Psychotherapy.* Hoboken: Wiley, 2001.

Diamond, Julie. *Power: A User's Guide.* Santa Fe: Belly Song Press, 2016.

DiAngelo, Robin. *White Fragility: Why It's So Hard for White People to Talk About Racism.* Boston: Beacon Press, 2018.

Dossey, Larry. *Space, Time & Medicine.* Boston: Shambala Publications Inc., 1982.

———. *Healing Words: The Power of Prayer and the Practice of Medicine.* New York: Harper Collins Publishers, 1993.

———. *One Mind: How Our Individual Mind Is Part of a Greater Consciousness and Why It Matters.* Carlsbad: Hay House Inc., 2014.

Frankl, Viktor. *Man's Search for Meaning. An Introduction to Logotherapy.* Boston: Beacon Press, 2006.

Gardner, Howard. *Intelligence Reframed: Multiple Intelligences for the 21st Century.* New York: Basic Books, 1999.

Gawande, Atul. *The Checklist Manifesto: How to Get Things Right.* New York: Metropolitan Books, 2010.

———. *Being Mortal: Medicine and What Matters in the End.* New York: Metropolitan Books, 2014.

Geller, Shari M. *A Practical Guide to Cultivating Therapeutic Presence.* Washington: American Psychological Association, 2017.

Gendlin, Eugene. *Focusing.* New York: Bantam Books [revised edition], 1981.

Goleman, Daniel. *Emotional Intelligence.* New York: Bantam Books, 1995.

Illich, Ivan. *Medical Nemesis.* London: Calder & Boyars, 1974.

Laing, Ronald David. *Wisdom, Madness and Folly: The Making of a Psychiatrist 1927–1957.* London: Macmillan, 1985.

Mann, Thomas. *The Coming Victory of Democracy.* New York: Alfred A. Knopf, Inc., 1938.

Marmot, Michael. *The Health Gap: The Challenge of an Unequal World.* London: Bloomsbury, 2015.

Marx, Karl. *The 18th Brumaire of Louis Bonaparte*. Cabin John: Wildside Press, 2008.

Mindell, Amy. *Metaskills: The Spiritual Art of Therapy*. Tempe: New Falcon, 1994/2001.

Mindell, Arnold. *Dreambody: The Body's Role in Revealing the Self*. London: Routledge & Kegan Paul, 1982.

Mindell, Arnold. *Sitting in the Fire: Large Group Transformation Using Conflict and Diversity*. Portland: Lao Tse Press, 1995.

———. *The Dreammaker's Apprentice: Using Heightened States of Consciousness to Interpret Dreams*. Charlottesville: Hampton Roads Publishing Company Inc., 2001.

———. *The Quantum Mind and Healing: How to Listen and Respond to your Body's Symptoms*. Charlottesville: Hampton Roads Publishing Company Inc., 2004.

———. *Process Mind: A User's Guide to Connecting to the Mind of God*. Wheaton: Quest Books, 2010.

———. *Conflict: Phases, Forums, and Solutions: For Our Dreams and Body, Organizations, Governments, and Planet*. Portland: World Tao Press, 2017.

Morin, Pierre, and Gary Reiss. *Inside Coma: A New View of Awareness, Healing, and Hope*. Santa Barbara: Praeger, 2010.

Morin, Pierre. *Health in Sickness, Sickness in Health*. Portland: Deep Democracy Exchange, 2014.

Nietzsche, Friedrich Wilhelm. *The Gay Science*. Minneola: Dover Publications, 2006.

Oluo, Ijeoma. *So You Want to Talk About Race*. New York: Seal Press, 2018.

Pollan, Michael. *Cooked: A Natural History of Transformation*. New York: Penguin Books, 2013.

Rinpoche, Chokyi Nyima, with David R. Shlim. *Medicine & Compassion: A Tibetan Lama's Guidance for Caregivers*. Somerville: Winston Publications, 2006.

Rumi, Jalal al-Din. *The Essential Rumi*, trans. Coleman Barks. San Francisco: Harper, 2004.

Sen, Amartya. *Development as Freedom*. New York: Alfred A. Knopf Inc., 1999.

Siegel, Daniel J. *The Developing Mind: How Relationships and the Brain Interact to Shape Who We Are, 2nd ed*. New York: The Guilford Press, 2012.

Solomon, Andrew. *Far from the Tree*. New York: Scribner, 2012.

Stenner, Karen. *The Authoritarian Dynamic*. Cambridge, England: Cambridge University Press, 2005.

Sweet, Victoria. *Slow Medicine: The Way to Healing*. New York: Riverhead Books, 2017.

Vaillant, George E. *Triumphs of Experience: The Men of the Harvard Grant Study*. Cambridge: Belknap Press, 2012.

Varela, F.J., E. Thompson, and E. Rosch. *The Embodied Mind: Cognitive Science and Human Experience*. Cambridge, Mass: MIT Press, 1991.

Van Sertima, Ivan (ed.). *Golden Age of the Moors*. Livingston: Transaction Publishers, 1992.

Von Franz, Marie-Louise. "The Process of Individuation," in *Man and His Symbols*, ed. Carl G. Jung. New York: Doubleday Publ., 1964.

Weil, Andrew. *Spontaneous Happiness: Step-by-Step to Peak Emotional Wellbeing*. New York: Little, Brown and Company, 2011.

INDEX

~2~

A

stillness, 106–107
stress, 116, 183–184
subjective experiences
  disenfranchisement of, 4, 72, 74
  exploring, 40, 47–48, 89
  insight from, 75–76
  value and meaning of, 15, 32
suffering
  caused by social dynamics, 105,
    108, 143, 160
  caused by trauma, 157
  empathy and compassion for,
    172, 184–187
  in illness experience, 99
  meaningful, 174, 186
  of providers, 144
symptoms
  communing with, 86–94
  dreaming of, 13–15
  exploration of, xx, 180
  meaning of, x, 36–38, 76, 174
synchronicity, 173
systemic oppression. *See* oppression

T

teeth grinding, 47
Tippett, Krista, 70, 106
traditional healing, 12
trauma
  health disparities and, 120–122
  health effects of, 22–23, 45–47,
    156–157
  Process-oriented approach, 7–9
  understanding, 186–187
  vicarious, 184
tribalism, 158–159
trusting relationships, 98–99,
  128–129, 185
Tweedy, Damon, 138–139

V

Varela, Francisco, 86
vicarious resilience, 185–186
victimhood and victimization, 8,
  27–28, 45, 99–100, 129, 186
von Franz, Marie Louise, 51, 174
Vosseler, Martin, xix

W

wealth distribution, 115
Western medicine, ix
  See also small medicine
white fragility, 158–163
Wilson, Margo, 114
wu wei, 177

ABOUT THE AUTHOR

PIERRE MORIN, MD, PHD, directs a community outpatient mental health clinic that serves refugees and trauma survivors in Portland, Oregon. A native of Switzerland, Dr. Morin began his career as a physician working in the fields of brain injury recovery and psychosocial medicine. He is co-author of *Inside Coma* and author of *Health in Sickness, Sickness in Health,* and has written numerous articles on mind-body medicine and community health. Dr. Morin is an international coach and trainer and the current co-president of the International Association of Process-Oriented Psychology (IAPOP).